The Bone Reporter

The Bone Reporter

In which the reader is encouraged to join the author in the
adventurous pursuit of his once-formidable potency.

Marshall Brinn

© 2017 Marshall Brinn
All rights reserved.

ISBN-13: 9781979491716
ISBN-10: 1979491712

For Amy, of course.

Acknowledgements

I WANT TO express my gratitude and appreciation to Dr. Andrew Wagner and Jodi Mechaber of Beth Israel Deaconess and Dr. Ravi Kacker and Kevin Flinn of the Boston Men's Health for their compassionate and excellent care. Heartfelt thanks to my intrepid band of first and insightful readers, Noah Efron, Joe Kruger, Phil Rosenblatt, Eilon Schwartz, Bill Slott, Josh Star-Lack, Alon Tal and Susan Warchaizer. Much love to my kids, Ayelet, Lior, and Sarah who have been great sources of support and love through this adventure. Finally, boundless love and gratitude to Amy for every moment contained in this book, and for every moment that precedes and follows it.

Two Months Out

1. Watching the Scoreboard

Let's just start with the fact that I lost my prostate and move on from there. Let's not focus on the details of how it got lost, who might have taken it, where it might be, whether it is well, or whether it misses me. The bottom line is this: I'm pretty sure it isn't coming back.

Okay, I didn't *lose* my prostate. It's not like I woke up one day, and it was gone. But that's the way people talk about it. "So," they would begin earnestly, "I understand you're losing your prostate."

"Yes," I would reply, "but I have prostate insurance and expect to be compensated royally."

In fact, my wife, Amy, and I were sitting in my urologist's office when we learned that my prostate and I would be parting ways. It was going to have to "go to a farm upstate"—I think those were his words, anyway. Who can remember?

There were scores involved. I'm a numbers guy, so this was right up my alley. First there was the Prostate-specific Antigen or PSA score, which we'd been monitoring for months. It should be present but low in men with healthy prostates. Mine was high, and getting higher. After hovering around two for most of my middle-aged life, it was suddenly in the sixes—not terribly high, but high. It was probably nothing. Or, if it was something, it was something else. But still, just be sure, there would be a biopsy. Just to, you know, rule things out.

To this point, we had all been playing by the same rules. No one mentions cancer, and everyone goes home happy. But the biopsy (which was mightily unpleasant, probably among the top ten worst things I experienced during the course of this whole sordid tale) begot the Gleason score, which ranks from 1 (low) to 5 (high) how abnormal the tissue is on either side of the prostate. Mine was "5 over 3, on both sides." (The "over" means most is "5" but most of the rest is "3"). I took issue with that right away: it didn't sound like a score to me at all. How can you tell who is winning? The urologist, however, was no longer in a joking mood. He said he was surprised. That this wasn't what he'd expected. And then, without warning, he broke the rules. This was cancer, and a highly "non-indolent"—his gentlemanly way of saying "aggressive"—form of it. The prostate would need to go. And soon.

2. Keeping It Dry

Most people, myself included until recently, have no idea what a prostate is or what it does. They know it is something that doctors use as an excuse to prod you. They know that as you get older, it grows and makes it harder to get a good hearty stream of pee going. They know that it can get cancerous. That's pretty much it. I always figured it was kind of like the appendix or the tonsils: nice to have it, but no big deal if you lose it. Turns out, not so much.

The first thing that my urologist explained to me was that the prostate is where semen is produced—and the average ejaculate is about 99 percent semen to 1 percent sperm. Any orgasm I had without the prostate would be "dry." I confess that this was enough to distract me for much of the rest of that visit. A dry orgasm? I wasn't in the market for a new variety: the current brand suited me just fine.

That said, I'd never thought of "wetness" as being one of the major benefits of an orgasm, especially now that my procreative years were behind me. Maybe dry wouldn't be so bad. Maybe it would feel exactly the same, just, you know, less ejaculate-y. Maybe it would be even *more* awesome, with all the energy my body had put into creating semen now focused solely on my own pleasure. You lose something, you gain something. That seemed only fair. Images of Richter-scale orgasms filled my head. This losing-my-prostate thing could be just fine, I told myself, just fine.

3. More Details are Revealed and Concealed

Some people don't know when to stop. My urologist could have just thrown the mike down at that moment and been a big hit. But he went on. Removing the prostate usually has two very prominent side effects:

1. You become incontinent.
2. You become impotent.

You may rest assured that he had my full attention. At this point, he started spouting a long series of medical Mad Libs:

Most men in your situation find that **REALLY, REALLY IMPORTANT BODILY FUNCTION** takes **SOME DEPRESSINGLY LARGE NUMBER** to **SOME EVEN MORE HORRIFYING NUMBER** months to mostly return. And even then, it isn't quite the same.

Did you notice all the qualifiers there?

Most men? I wondered. *Am I like most men*? Or was I somehow better and thus able to avoid these two fates entirely? Would I overcome them in a matter of days and be good as new? Or what if I were somehow lesser and *never* regained my faculties?

What was with all the time ranges, anyway? Three to twelve months for bladder control? Twelve to thirty-six for erections? These were margins of error you could drive a truck through—though not a penis, apparently. And just what did "not quite the same" mean? I suspected he was hinting at "different—and not better." I could imagine what it meant to have no bladder control. Or no erection. I dreaded it, but I could imagine it. But what did it mean to have a different kind of bladder control? A new form of erection? The mind boggles.

And again, on that last one: *it isn't quite the same.* He didn't say, "For some, men it often isn't quite the same." A whole paragraph of weasel wording, and all of a sudden one thing he's sure of. After the whole period of working through an unknown amount of time, effort, and uncertain prospects, the only thing you can be certain of is that you won't be back where you started. I was silent. My wife was too. I know she had a lot of questions, but she probably felt that it was my dick, so I got the floor.

He continued. "I realize this is a lot to take in. Let it sink in, talk things over with your wife. Don't worry—we'll go over it all again when I see you again."

"After surgery," he added.

4. Introduction

This little journal, which I'm calling the *Boner Report*, is about my assault on detail number two above—and, I suppose, its assault on me. It's my report on what we refer to as "sexual function" (in doctor's pamphlets) or "getting it up" (just about anywhere else). I've been at this now for eight weeks. I'm "eight weeks out," as they call it, which means "eight weeks since the prostate was taken out," but which I hear as "eight weeks since your flame was extinguished." I can say this. I am hopeful. There is some reason for hope. But hope by its nature is not reasonable, so be prepared for however this may go down.

On those last few words: I find that inadvertent sexual innuendo has infested my writing. I make no apologies. At least my pen is hard and has some ink in it...And yes, I'm actually typing on a flat and unaroused computer keyboard. This seems fitting to me.

5. Not the Boner Report

By the way, I don't want to spend your time or mine talking about all the pee stuff. It isn't fun, but it isn't great drama either. With patience, it pretty much comes back. At least it has for me, so far. As I write this, eight weeks out, I am fully in control of my bladder except when I sneeze, cough, hiccup, laugh, or make sudden movements. Which, my wife tells me, puts me in the camp with every woman who has ever given birth. So I hoard my sympathy points for where it counts and grin and bear it on this one.

That said, there is a surprising connection between these two functions—surprising to me, anyway. I had always thought of peeing and coming as completely separate things, confident that there was a solid switch between these two rails.

I was right, but that switch was the prostate (or one of the things nearby that gets removed with it). So we may need to take a few steps in the yellow snow as we walk down this (maybe someday) straight and (maybe someday not) narrow path.

6. No Action

I know most men claim never to have problems getting it up. It's a standard macho defense mechanism, probably wired down in our lizard brains. But for me, up until this surgery, it was true: I never had a problem with erections. Not as an adult, anyway.

Back in junior high and high school, I had plenty of erection problems. An innuendo in a movie, a smile from a girl, just sitting in certain positions would awaken the snake, sometimes quickly. It was always embarrassing, and you'd have to do your best to adjust your package in as nonchalant a way as possible. These adjustments never, somehow, went unnoticed by my peer group.

So, yes, that was a problem. But the opposite problem is one I don't think I've had. Maybe I did a few times and blocked it out. I have some memory of being too drunk a few times and finding it difficult to proceed (I first said "hard" there, but I think you'll agree it would have been the wrong word choice). But mostly my erection was there without much coaxing when summoned to duty.

I always awoke with the classic Morning Boner. I often awoke in the middle of the night ready to impale something in my dreams and needing to position myself with care to get back to sleep. I will fess up to this, though. From around age forty-five or so (maybe forty, maybe fifty) my erections would occasionally not be as hard as I'd like. Or as durable. I could get it up, get it in, and then it would kinda slip out, or just not have the oomph that the occasion called for. Usually, with a little attention and concentration, my wife and I could summon the sacred blood flows to their mystic channels and all would be well. But this was new, and a little unsettling.

That said, this is new territory for me. What I have now is dead wood. Entirely dead. No amount of coaxing, stimulation, concentration, or prayer can result in even the slightest amount of engorgement. No action. All systems are stop.

7. What That's Like?

It sucks—that's what it's like. Can't believe you even asked.

First, it's surreal. It has a dreamlike quality. It is so strange and unfamiliar that it makes the whole day-to-day experience of life assume a Twilight Zone quality.

Second, it is infuriating. Sexual arousal is one of the basic functions included in the contract between you and your body. I feel betrayed and cheated. I did my part—didn't I? Did I fail to participate in some critical prostate-health exercise or diet regimen of which I was unaware? Who said you could stop doing yours?

Third, it is scary. If your boner can up and leave, what is safe?

Finally, it is humbling. Face it, I never did anything to bring about my potency: it was a gift. Now the gift has been recalled. What else have I taken unearned credit for?

8. Prospects

I mentioned that my urologist said that most men got some "function" back within one to three years, which is like saying nothing at all. He did provide some other information, none of which adds up to a realistic forecast.

On one hand, I'm young (ish) and (otherwise) healthy and in (pretty) good shape. So I should be able to recover pretty quickly. In fact, my recovery from the surgery itself was pretty remarkable: I was back at work in three weeks.

On another hand, the surgery was pretty radical. They needed to cut out not just the prostate but some of the surrounding tissue and nerves (out of caution that the cancer might have spread) as well. And these nerves, lo and behold, are the ones that control the building of the Eiffel Tower. The very same ones. What a cruel twist of anatomical design.

An important factor, then, is how many of these nerves are left intact. If they're all there, no problem: boner city. If they're all cut out, no more erections, full stop. Most men fall in some hazy middle ground. Some nerves get removed, others remain. Whether these are the right nerves or provide a critical mass, no one knows.

So after the surgery, my urologist and nurse practitioner both came in and visited me. They talked about how well the surgery had gone, told me that they thought they'd gotten it all. I confess that I hadn't even thought about that. *Of course* they got it all. That's what the surgery was *for*. It didn't occur to me that they might open me up and find all kinds of shit that weren't on their cut plan. I was worried about what *else* they'd gotten.

I asked about the nerves and how much they'd been able to "spare." Yep, that's the language: nerve-sparing surgery. Like Isaac on the altar, about to be sliced to smithereens, and then a voice comes and spares him from his awful fate.

"We were able to save some," the urologist answered.

"So that's good," the practitioner added.

"So I'll be able to…" I coached them.

"There's a chance," they both answered, practically in unison.

I've played that moment in my mind over and over these last two months. *There's a chance.* That means it is not impossible. But that they have no way of quantifying it. Could be. Could not be. Both completely reasonable outcomes, and no way to tell which is more likely. In fact, the most likely is some middle outcome. Weak erections. Erratic erections. Short-lived erections. There's a chance. But what chance? And of what?

This is where I am at the moment. There is nothing happening down-stairs. Actually, that isn't entirely true. I'll elaborate in a bit. But in general, it's all quiet on the southern front. "Be patient," my practitioner counsels. It takes a long time. But again, no one knows how long, or where I'll be at the end.

I'm not sure I've ever been in a situation with so much uncertainty. I suppose the cancer itself had this quality (it was also couched in terms of probabilities and timelines and demographic distributions). But the whole detection-to-extraction cycle was so quick (weeks) that I never had much time to ponder it. With this one, I've got nothing but time. Heaven willing, of course.

9. Little Blue Pill

The nurse practitioner, Jodi, recommended that I start taking Viagra after about four weeks. She said it was good to keep the blood vessels in the penis from atrophying. I couldn't agree more. But she cautioned that I probably wouldn't be able to get an erection for a while even with medi-cation. In fact, if the wrong set of nerves had been removed, no amount of Viagra would help. So I've been taking Viagra once a week. A blue pill, much like you see on commercials.

My sex life with Amy is none of your goddamn business. We have had a very good sex life, especially (oddly, or perhaps not) in our middle age. I'm fine with sharing the details of my half of the equation, but her half or the whole we create together I'm keeping private. That's all I'll say. Seriously, back off. But we're very much a team as we navigate this little obstacle course, trying to recreate old favorites in new ways or create new things that work. And, of course, there are a lot of wonderful things in a sexual relationship that don't require erections. Check and check.

One of the pamphlets Jodi gave me as we were discharged from the hospital informed me that physical stimulation was much more effective than "imagery stimulation" at my stage of things. I found this strange. In my previous experience, getting a hard-on was almost completely about imagery stimulation: The anticipation of sex. The talking about sex. The fantasizing about sex. This was the stuff that brought the eel out from the briny depths. Physical stimulation was what led to later stages, like arousal and orgasm.

Indeed, though, imagery stimulation of any sort has been of no help in getting an erection. Getting excited, sure. But hard, no. And at this point, even physical stimulation has had only limited results. On a very good (perhaps deluded with wishful thinking) day, Amy and I have convinced ourselves that there is some slight swelling. Some enlargement. Nothing that you'd call an erection. It's not HARD. Not even stiff. Just maybe a little less of a wallflower. Maybe that's something. Maybe that's encouraging. Maybe that's step one of a long journey. Maybe that's the whole path. No one knows.

Does the Viagra help? I think maybe so. From my purely scientific studies of stimulation without Viagra, I can discern no flow of blood at all. And with the Viagra (one hour later, empty stomach) I can feel a lot of heaviness in the groin area, the balls, the muscles behind the penis. Like something is going on down there. Like someone is trying desperately to find the "ON switch." But so far, whoever it is hasn't found it.

10. If You had to Choose

A little anatomy trivia for your reading pleasure. You can have erections without orgasms. And you can have orgasms without erections. They are entirely different mechanisms. Erections are a nerve response, as we've discussed. Orgasms are a muscle spasm—who knew?

A year or so ago, I was on a particular antidepressant for a while. I couldn't have an orgasm to save my life (which seems like a great premise for a combo romantic comedy and adventure thriller). Amy and I would wind up sore and exhausted (or I on my own, again, strictly in the name of science). No frigging orgasm. The washing machine just wouldn't shift into rinse cycle. Like there was a short in the circuitry somewhere. Trust me, this was not a great situation.

So let me pose it to you: Which is worse, erection without orgasm? Or orgasm without erection? To answer that question, you need to imagine what it's like to have an orgasm without an erection. To my surprise, I learned that it's pretty much like a regular orgasm in terms of feeling, intensity, and sleepiness afterward.

Imagine maniacally milking a cow—or, to be precise, one teat. Imagine massaging a quarter-full sausage casing, or perhaps rhythmically stroking a celery stalk freshly fetched from a pot of soup. All for a very long time. That should give you a rough idea. So, which would you prefer: straw with no shake, or shake with no straw? "I want both" is an unacceptable answer.

To me, this quandary gets right to the root (sorry) of the question of what sex is and what's pleasurable about it. An orgasm is a great thing—one of the best things the human body can do, I'd venture. But an erection allows you to have intercourse. To penetrate. To thrust. To give that kind of pleasure to someone else, to have unparalleled intimacy with someone else. I miss that terribly.

Plus (and this is the weird Freudian or maybe Jungian stuff) there's just something about having an erection. It's not just that it makes you feel like a man (though, sure, it does). It makes you feel alive. It makes you feel like someone who can create, who can DO, who can BE, who IS. It is a statement of identity (albeit concealed carry, ideally).

Fundamentally, one is about giving and the other is about receiving. Sex is made up of both of these. Frankly, the most important part of sex, the part I truly wouldn't want to live without, is intimacy—breaking down walls and flowing together with someone else. Not being alone inside your own little fortress. That's the greatest pleasure. And if these images of castles evoke images of battering rams, so be it.

11. To Die for

Just a little aside. I remember joking before the surgery (when I really thought that all of this would be fine and provide no disruption to my awesome mojo) that I'd rather die than not be able to have an erection.

Honestly, I think a number of men have put off their prostate surgery (taking a wait-and-see approach or not even consulting with surgeons) because of this fear. For the record, I was joking, I'd rather live. Good trade-off, no regrets.

12. Blame the Vagina

I went through a period a few days ago where I couldn't stop wondering why the vagina needed to be so tight. If it were a little more loose or gaping, I could enter without needing to be *so* erect. I mean, what gives? The ravings of the erection-starved, admittedly. When you have an erection, the tightness is part of the magic. I know that. Usually.

13. Nocturnal Admissions

Two things about sleeping. First, I wonder if I have hard-ons in my sleep. Maybe they come back first in sleep, and that's a sign that they're on their way back in prime time. I'm not sure how to tell, though. I saw a movie once about someone tying a hair around his shaft and see if it broke during the night. But I might have made that up. And the idea of tying a hair around the shaft of my dick made it difficult to breathe.

Second, I find that I'm dreaming of *having* an erection all the time. This is very different from a sex dream, or even a sex dream in which my erection figures prominently. I am not having sex dreams so far as I can recall. (And which is the chicken and which the egg? Does my dream center know that there's no boner, so nothing R-rated or beyond?). These are dreams about having an erection.

A few nights ago, I dreamed that my wife and I were on the beach, and my erection came out of my swimming trunks. Everyone on the beach came by and congratulated me. Last night, a group of paparazzi flooded the media with images of my impressive elevation. In another dream, my erection was a float in a parade—not *honored* with a float (though that would be cool too); it *was* the float. These dreams probably mean something, though what I can't imagine.

14. Stirrings

My surgery was already a good couple of months ago. But the internal FEMA project is not yet complete. There's a lot of innards vying for the space once occupied by my prostate. Lots of sutures in various states of dissolve. Lots of nerves hanging loosely like power lines among downed trees. So, when I am sitting quietly, particularly attentive to my body, I feel lots of activity. Zaps, pings, pressures, aches, static on the nervous system radio station.

Maybe this is just the way it will always be. Stuff jangling around. But sometimes (at my most optimistic) I wonder if this isn't the experience of potency coming back to life. Of wires being reattached and leaks being patched. Of circuits being slowly powered back on. I feel these all the time, and that kind of hope follows in an instant.

More: occasionally, on the couch, I feel something that feels like the early onset of a hard-on. You know how it works. There are a few tentative little tingles, maybe the head, the shaft, the balls. Maybe you don't quite know where. And then, like a charmed snake, it starts to come to life, squirming around in a confined dark space (my underwear, duh). In the past, this would have been my cue to break it—oh, what I'd give for one of those misbegotten boners I have broken into submission!— or shift it to a more comfortable and inconspicuous position. Or, if it's actually "go time," let it out and onward and (especially) upward. But for now, it is just disembodied sensation, not unlike the proverbial phantom limb.

15. Bonerian Logic

I've been thinking a lot of the state of the erection over the course of my life. When I was young, it appeared at the most inopportune times. Now it fails to appear at the most opportune times. As a computer scientist and thus a poor man's logician, I visualize the problem as a logic diagram. What circumstances cross the having/not-having against the wanting/not wanting of an erection?

	Having	Not Having
Wanting	(A)	(C)
Not Wanting	(B)	(D)

(A) and (D) are flip-sides of the ideal coin. You have it when you want it, you don't have it when you don't. Perfect alignment. Thoroughly unachievable over the course of our lifetimes, at least reliably or for very long. But mostly I fell into these boxes in the 1980s–2000s. Good times. (B) is me in the early 1970s: not wanting an erection (not even having the slightest idea what to do with one) and yet getting them, and plentifully. (C) is me in the 2010s, wanting an erection and not getting one.

To me, this feels like a looking-glass distortion of the old chestnut about regressing to your youth as you age, but in ways that are flipped and cross-wired. Lewis Carroll would have been amused, if he weren't so preoccupied with prepubescent girls.

16. The Best Distraction Ever

The period between the diagnosis and the surgery is a blur. I think there are several reasons for this. First, it was all very quick. All told, it was only five weeks from "gotta go" to "gone." Second, the entire period was covered with a thick fog of uncertainty, fear, and denial. Most importantly, I was busy trying on suits and writing toasts. My son's wedding was scheduled smack in the middle of this period, two weeks after the diagnosis and three weeks before the surgery. Most of my energy, emotional and otherwise, was focused on the big day and all that surrounded it. Amy's too.

The wedding was just wonderful. I'll spare you a recitation of who wore what or my impressions of the caterer, the band, or the flowers. Amy and I were in California (where our son and now daughter-in-law live) for ten days, frantically meeting new relatives, hanging with our own relatives and friends who made the trek, and celebrating with abandon. Trust me, it was a great joy, start to finish.

I do want to share with you one moment that bears on our topic. The day of the wedding, maybe three hours before the processional, my son and I and his five or six sundry groomsmen and attendants found ourselves in a hotel room watching football. We were waiting for the photographer to come and take some fake-spontaneous pictures of him getting dressed, me helping him with his tie, that sort of thing.

I knew his friends from years of carpooling—dropping them off at dances, picking them up from games, housing them for weekend sleepovers. I hadn't seen most of them in nearly a decade: boys to men. One of them, it turned out, was now a medical statistician, fluent in various diseases and how they tend to play out. I asked him about it with great interest. "I understand you have some surgery coming up," he told me. I didn't realize my son had shared this with him. I didn't mind; I just didn't think it was something he'd mention to his friends. I was touched that he had.

I talked about the diagnosis. I shared my scores, which his friend ate up. He knew just what PSA trajectories and Gleason scores meant, better than I. I hinted at the potential challenges that lay ahead, though I downplayed them through hedges of "you never know," and "hopefully." The room got quiet (the game was already on mute). Everyone wanted to hear.

These were men just at the start of their roads of virility, still looking for love or just having found it. None had yet had kids. All were starting to traverse the beautiful wilderness that is sex between loving partners. They had their full potency and then some. Their libidos overflowing. They were me, some thirty years ago.

I measured the distance between them and me, and I could sense that they were doing the same. We were taking measure of what might lie ahead for me—and, some day, for them. The fleetingness of love and life, there on this day full of both, hung in the air. Nice job, Downer Dad. Then the photographer came and brought us back to the present.

After the wedding, they each gave me a big hug and wishes of good luck. I hugged back tightly.

17. Dedicated to Mrs. Reitz, whom I Despised

When I was in third grade, I was—apparently—a terror. I don't remember this exactly, but I do have my report cards from that year, which refer to conferences my parents attended. Mrs. Reitz's last entry, scribbled on my June report card, read, "I'm afraid little progress has been made on which I can report." Mrs. Reitz died aboard a cruise ship when I was in college (my parents sent me the clipping). I felt a little more pleasure than I should have. Perhaps that's why I'm in the boat I am in now. Who knows?

In any event, I'll sign off this installment of the *Boner Report* echoing her admonishment—but fully aware of all the growth and change and achievement that lay ahead of me when she wrote it: I'm afraid little progress has been made on which I can report.

Three Months Out

1. First Things First

WE SAW MY urologist several weeks ago, at the three-month anniversary of the surgery. By his accounting, all is going well. He's mostly interested in the cancer-y part of things, and on that front, I'm pleased to say, things are nice and quiet. My PSA score is zero, which means none of the nasty cells seem to have colonized in foreign, non-prostate territories. All good.

I'm to see my urologist again in nine months, one year from the surgery. I'll have PSA tests every three months, then every six, then eventually (if they stay at zero) annually. I felt a little surprised. That's it? I see him once after three months, and then I'm on my own for another nine? Just routine check-ins and maintenance from now on; he's got other people to worry about. I suppose this a good thing. But I did like the feeling that there was someone actively looking at my case and how things were progressing.

He asked how I was doing with continence (pretty good) and erections (not so good). He counseled patience, advising me that potency usually takes about three years to get to "wherever you're going to get to." Put one way, you don't know what kind of function you'll have until three years have passed. Put another way, whatever is happening by three years, that's pretty much the show. I'm only three months into a three-year process. Patience, jackass, patience. Remember that joke from middle school? While he was willing to answer my questions, he was clearly eager to pass the whole "lifestyle" recovery on to someone else. As we were leaving, he gave me a referral to someone in his practice specializing in "male sexual function." One wonders how you get into that particular specialty.

2. The Options

Essentially, my urologist spelled out these basic options for recovering potency:

a. *Patience.* Wait long enough, and it comes back by itself. Nerves heal, blood superhighways reopen, brain and body get time to reacquaint with one another. This is the preferred option if it works out, but it's not common. Even after waiting a full three years.

b. *Viagra and friends.* This is a common solution. Men often respond well to Viagra after prostatectomies, and that does the trick. It hasn't so much for me, so far, but maybe it will over time—who knows?

c. *Suppositories.* Wait, what? Apparently there is a "penile suppository" that dilates the blood vessels in the penis, causing blood to flow and an erection to develop. No nerves involved. It works for about 40 percent of men. But let's step back for a second. My experience with suppositories has been limited to putting them up my ass for hemorrhoids or constipation. They're fairly big things that need to be pushed in pretty far. How the hell does this work with a penile suppository? I think I speak for most men when I point out that the hole isn't very big. I'm intrigued—maybe it's a hair-thin suppository that goes in easily and painlessly?—but pretty skeptical.

d. *Injection.* Again, what? Yep, if the suppository doesn't work, apparently there's an injection you can shoot directly into the shaft of your penis, and it will give you an erection. It's the same basic chemical as the suppository, and it works for like 95 percent of men who are willing to stick themselves in the dick with a syringe. Which is apparently around zero percent. My doctor said this was the option he would choose if it were up to him, "but I'm used to dealing with syringes and penises." I didn't consider this comforting. I can just imagine the steamy narrative. Man and woman are getting hot and heavy. Man retires to the restroom "I'll be right back…don't you move!." He goes to the bathroom, a blood-curdling scream is heard, followed by the sound of someone's head beating against the wall and twenty minutes of moaning and sobbing. Then he returns, fully erect, but bloody or bandaged: "Now then, where were we?"

e. *Pumps.* No, not the high-heel kind. We're talking about penis pumps. Insert penis, pump as one would a bicycle tire, and voila, stiffness ensues. I have no idea how much pumping is required, nor how solid or long-lasting the effect. I was, however, struck by the nurse practitioner's breezy way of describing how one acquires one of these. "Oh, you can get them at novelty shops, or online at special websites." We had now pierced the membrane separating medical supplies and sex toys. Novelty shops? Where one might buy fake vomit or whoopee cushions? Try again: penis pumps are the kind of thing one buys next to the dildos and blow-up dolls in sex shops (or equally shady websites).

   They are the kind of thing that makes for great punchlines in movies: they are discovered at airport security; hilarity ensues when one, say, overpumps…I'm not saying these things don't work, nor that I wouldn't be game to trying if it seemed like the next natural option. But unlike these other options, no one at a respectable hospital is going to be writing you a prescription for one.

f. *Implants.* Yep, the last station on this gruesome track is the implant. I don't know much about this and hope I never do. But the idea is that metal or hard plastic is surgically implanted in the shaft of the penis, and through some action (magnets? remote control? dialing a special number? tweeting @mydick?) the implant elongates to the point of firmness. Then, after use, the erector set is dismantled, presumably by the opposite means. This seems pretty amazing to me, even worse than the shot. But I have a friend who says his father-in-law, a man somewhere in his early eighties, needed to have his implant replaced because he had "worn it out." That man is a hero to me.

g. *The default option*. The final, unspoken option, is nothing. Just kind of accept that this lack of potency is a fact of life and give up on trying to make it better. I've been reading a lot of blogs recently with lots of different people writing about their experiences. And not a small number of them just ended up saying, "I gave up—it's just not worth it." It's difficult to imagine coming to that conclusion. But I am at the start of what is likely to be a very long and frustrating path.

3. Four Hours

Oh, my doctor mentioned one other thing, almost in passing. When you are bypassing the natural pathways of erection, there really is a possibility that the erection won't go down. Normally, after you have an orgasm, the same nerves that crank up the cannon start to crank it down. But with these various Rube Goldberg schemes, there isn't anyone listening for the orgasm signal. So the thing people make fun of in Viagra commercials—"Call your doctor if you have an erection lasting more than four hours"—is a real thing. If your body doesn't know how to make one, it only makes sense that it might not know how to unmake one. And having a perpetual erection, besides the obvious being-in-public challenges, can be bad for your poor penis (something about blood pooling, cellular fatigue, things I can imagine but only if I'm not required to stay in the realm of science). Anyway, it's a thing. Something else to keep in mind.

4. Dry My Ass

One thing my original urologist mentioned to me at the very beginning was that after a prostatectomy, orgasms would be "dry." He meant no semen. And he's right on that front. But I gotta say this is one of the weirdest and most bewildering aspects of this whole process. Instead of shutting off the flow of urine, as they have all my life, orgasms now open it up. I have to pee a lot in the course of a sexual encounter, which—as you can imagine—is a bit of a mood breaker. And orgasm, unless you are amazingly attentive to emptying the bladder literally moments before the big moment, is full of urine. Urine flowing out with the force and velocity formerly reserved for semen. It is not a pretty sight, and it means you need lots of towels, old tee-shirts, rags, what have you, to contain the flood.

This is one of those things that my doctor assures me improves over time "as you get to know your body again." But it does seem like a difficult thing to overcome (sorry for the pun) or master (sorry for the slightly more subliminal pun).

5. Condoms

I mentioned this to my doctor, the whole pee and sex thing. It seemed like a topic one might bring up with one's urologist. Aside from his usual counseling patience thing, he mentioned that if we wanted to have oral sex (the receiving kind, that is) I should wear a condom. This makes all the sense in the world, except for one small thing. How do you put on a condom if you can't get an erection? I asked him, and he admitted that it was a bit of a catch-22. Usually I would be pleased to win debating points like this, but somehow this exchange didn't feel very gratifying. My guess is that he's not that used to men trying to have sex without the erection being reinstated. But his suggestion also tells me that the urine-and-sex thing isn't going to go away when erections are back in the mix.

6. Definitions

The day before the appointment, the nurse practitioner had asked me if my wife and I had had intercourse. I confess I'm still not used to living in a world in which relative strangers are free to ask me questions like that. But even aside from that, it had become a very hard question to answer. I found myself getting very definitional and legalistic. What counts as intercourse? How much needs to be in for how long? I tried to adjust the definitions so that the answer would be "yes." Perhaps rubbing the head of the penis in the general area of the vagina was good enough?

She listened patiently and then said, "I think you'd know it if you had it." And fair enough. By the definition that I would have applied only a few months ago, no, we haven't. And no amount of redefining or contractual weasel-wording can make it feel that we have. We're trying. Mightily, I might say. That's something. But it's not enough to check the box on the nurse practitioner's form.

7. The Universal Solution

Both my nurse practitioner and my urologist have one piece of advice that they never fail to dispense for problems with urination or erection or orgasm: "Are you doing your Kegels?" They offer these as the solution to any problem. What's a Kegel, you say? It is a contraction of the pelvic floor. It's something you probably already do to hold in urine, or push that last little bit out. But in order to restore function after a prostatectomy, one is supposed to do something like ten at a time, five times a day. Which is really nothing. You can do them any time you want—sitting in meetings, trying to wake up, eating a meal…

I went through a period of doing these intensely: ten or twenty times more than they suggested. If a little Kegeling is good, a lot of Kegeling must be great! I'll be fixed in no time! Alas, it doesn't work that way, and (apparently) you can get Kegel fatigue so that your pelvic floor muscles don't want to respond on demand—they're spent, poor things. Or they can get so exercised that they stay in "on" position and don't easily turn back off.

To be specific, you're supposed to do Kegels while urinating. Start the flow, then stop it for five seconds, then let it start, then stop it. Repeat until bladder is empty. My problem was that I'd been doing so many Kegels that I would start the stream, stop it, and then it wouldn't turn back on. I'd feel the need to pee, but no pee would come out. I'd need to contract my abs to push the pee out. Which isn't the way it is supposed to work.

So I've put this magic wonder regimen on the back burner for a while, only doing them when I remember. Just what I need: another exercise regime to which I can be disloyal.

8. Dirty Talk

OK, if you're up for it, there's something very funny about trying to have intercourse, real honest-to-goodness intercourse, when you don't have an erection. Consider the usual kind of passionate exchange among couples in the throes of passion, saying things like "you're so deep in me," and "it's so big," and "it feels so good to be inside you." That sort of thing. I'm not quoting anything verbatim, mind you. And I know that people say things that may capture the feeling of the moment and not some objective reality (the "it's so big" part—who am I to judge?). But still and all, that's the kind of thing people say in the right circumstances. I've heard tell.

The current circumstance supplies its own kind of discourse: "is it in?" or "oops, it slipped out, let me try again," or "do you feel anything?." Like I said, it's funny. Though less so in the moment.

9. What Happens to the Sperm?

I think I mentioned that after the prostatectomy, the plumbing connecting the testicles, the foundries of sperm, and the penis are forever severed. But sperm is still created, and it still exits the balls. And then, like an astronaut on a space-walk whose line gets cut, it just floats around in the protoplasm. My doctor says the cells eventually just get re-absorbed back into the body. Yuck, sez I.

There is something you feel. When you have an orgasm, you feel it in your balls. They've done their job. They've produced the awesome head-and-tail delivery system of reproduction, in mass quantities. But they don't have the pleasure of feeling their creations going out to meet the world. All of this is a roundabout way of saying two words. Blue balls. They kind of ache after orgasm. Perhaps they're just expressing their emotions—which, I'm told, is a good thing from time to time.

10: Pin Pricks

Lately I've been feeling a lot of electric shocks in my penile area. Or perhaps they're more like a bee sting. Or maybe not quite that painful. But this is an area that has been pretty pampered through much of its life, so it tends to exaggerate. My immediate response is to believe that this is the feeling of long-hibernating nerves reawakening, or perhaps long-severed nerves reconnecting, or growing, or whatever the fuck nerves do. That this is the sign of something coming back to life.

My secondary response is that this is one of those things the doctors forget to tell you about: *Oh yes, you won't be able to get an erection. And you'll have periodic shocks in your dick from now on.* But you didn't hear that second one, because you stopped listening after the first. My next response was to think that it was all psychosomatic, my brain sending pings in hope of getting some echo from the wreck. Mostly I just cycle between these responses.

There: I just had one. As I was typing that last paragraph. Right as I was typing the word "cycle." Maybe it's got some Ouija-board quality that I can use to discern hidden truths by noting the words I'm typing when they happen.

11. Mark your Calendars

Dear reader, you've been patient. You've read that whole first collection and now all the entries in this one. Don't you deserve a little action? Well, action you shall have. We did it. Honest to goodness. No legalistic, technical definitions required. The real thing. Perhaps not my best performance ever. But real intercourse.

As noted, none of this is your damn business. But here's what I can tell you. I worked out Saturday morning. Blood pumping, energy high, perhaps testosterone too. Dunno. Nothing to eat or drink that morning. Bladder empty. Some forty minutes after taking a pill, and lots of stimulation of all types and from all sides and angles, I noticed that the head and maybe the top inch was somewhat swollen. If I took my hand and shmooshed it all up to the top, like you might with a half-deflated balloon, there was an actual hard, swollen (though tiny) erection on top of a flaccid pedestal. But this was something.

I'll refrain from describing the positions involved. But use your best engineer's sense of gravity and hydraulics. A lot of lube at the entrance, and I was able to push this head in. Then, in the instant after actual penetration, the whole penis woke up. Pow! I was in, I was deep, I was able to move in and out. No falling out. This was actual penetration, thrusting, the whole deal. We were both kind of speechless. We were even able to transition to other (less gravitationally and hydraulically sound) positions, and all was well.

I was not able to have an orgasm, though we worked at it pretty hard. I think that may be a ways off. Too much lube? Not enough friction? Nerves not really playing ball yet? Who knows. But don't get me wrong. It felt really good. The way sex feels: that kind of good. It felt miraculous. I literally didn't expect to have an experience like this so soon (or, on darker days, ever again). But there it was, just out of the blue. We were both pretty in-the-clouds the rest of the weekend.

12. And Yet, Not So Fast

The week after, a complete repeat performance. Same success. Same thrill. It seemed like a new sustainable achievement. A new platform on which to stand sturdily. Then, yesterday, we tried again. Nothing doing. No erection of any sort. Certainly not enough to achieve even the slightest penetration. The post-prostatectomy gods are cruel and capricious. Two steps forward, one step back. But still, I'll take it. Okay, enough for this installment. I'll sign off here and leave our hero dangling until next time.

You see what I did there, right?

Six Months Out

1. A Day to Remember

THIS EDITION OF the *Boner Report* all takes place on a single day. May 1. May Day. The International Day of Worker Solidarity and Dancing around Poles. And yes, there was some labor involved. I got to work (this is not the labor part), and there was an e-mail from the "Men's Health Clinic" that I had an appointment at 10:15 a.m. I had completely forgotten. Wasn't even in my calendar.

After reading the reminder, I remembered that this was really two appointments: one with a nurse practitioner to "take some measurements," and one with the doctor to go over them. Something about blood flow, if I recall. It all sounded pretty innocuous. I wondered why I might have blocked it out.

2. Men's Health Clinic

I got to my appointment with time to spare. It was close to my home, though I came from work. Had I remembered, I might have worked from home (or, if you prefer, "worked from home") that morning. But whatever.

I was actually quite curious about what a men's health clinic would be like. A clinic, I imagined, devoted to issues that were wholly male. Man issues. Y-chromosome issues. I imagined one wing devoted to baldness, another to troubling ear and nose hair, another to resolving long-simmering father/son issues. Nah. It's all about dick stuff.

I filled out a questionnaire about sexual performance and urinary performance—two topics at the very top of my list. I was pleased to be able to calculate my USS (urination satisfaction score) and find it was very high. It's been six months, and I really have very little to complain about on that front. And getting high scores on just about anything is what gets me out of bed in the morning.

The ED (oh come on, you know what ED stands for) score wasn't as gratifying. It was low. Very low. Which was why I was there—to do something about raising the score, and the mast it represented.

3. Why I Might Have Blocked It Out

I got called into the examining room. The NP, Kevin, was a nice guy—middle-aged, friendly, thick Boston accent. There was some kind of sonogram contraption on one side, with a screen and a bottle of goop. It seemed to me that what they were going to do was like they do for pregnant women: apply the goop and get a good picture of what was going on inside. This turned out to be mostly right. Except he wasn't trying to look inside but rather measure the strength of my blood flow, in and out. He wanted to make graphs (which, again, is my bread and butter).

But he had to take these measurements not on my penis as it was, but in its most aspirational and ennobled state. In short, he needed me to get an erection in order to measure why I couldn't get an erection. That's when I looked at the other side of the room and saw a set of vials and syringes.

He told me he was going to inject me with a dilation formulation, something that makes the blood vessels in the penis expand and would, we hoped, lead to an erection. I was a little horrified (I'd been a biter at the doctor's office as a kid) but also kind of fascinated. What would it feel like? And (more importantly) would it work?

Kevin explained that the intent was to use the shots, which I'd learn to self-administer if they were effective, until the nerves had healed enough to work on their own. It was intended as a station on the road to recovery, not the end of the line. Though for some people it is. Personally, if it worked and I could get used to giving myself the shots, I wasn't closing any doors.

So I took down my pants, and he inserted the syringe and emptied its contents inside. Did it hurt? Not really. The needle was extremely thin. The dilation chemicals burned a little as they filled the penis, but only for maybe two seconds. Then, I figured, I would wait for the magic.

4. Helping Things Along

Kevin said, "I'm going to give you ten minutes of privacy. I want you to work at getting the best erection you can. Really work at it. But don't go too far, if you know what I mean." I knew what he meant. "I'm sorry, I only have a couple of *Playboy*s here, I hope that'll do the trick." He pulled two somewhat worn copies of *Playboy* out of a drawer and put them on a table on my left. "I'll be back in ten minutes," he said, closing the door firmly behind him.

5. Really?

I loved his apology: "I only have a couple of *Playboy*s." As if he really owed me more and better stuff. My first response was kind of bemused shock. *Playboy*? What if I was aroused only by bondage-related double-penetration geriatric erotica? Or, more to the point, gay?

They apparently wanted me to use the *Playboy*s to help stroke my way to an erection. Hell, there was a computer just two feet away from me. Why not just let patients go wild online and clear the browser history when they're done? But in my normal postoperative state, no amount of "visual stimulation" (*Playboy* or otherwise) could produce the slightest swelling. So I was skeptical.

6. Playboy

Now I imagine some of my readers may be wondering just what *Playboy* is like. Like me, you may not have paged through an issue since your middle teens. So as a service to you, my readers, I decided to look through the issues. It is one weird magazine.

First, there are all these not-exactly-funny cartoons full of sexy women of exaggerated proportions. They often depict one of two situations. In one, a man and woman having sex are interrupted by his wife/girlfriend. "Go back to sleep," the man quips, "let's talk about this in the morning"—or something witty like that. In the second, a beautiful and—maybe—incredibly horny woman produces a jaw-dropping double entendre: "my pussy is hungry," said one, a cat at her feet. See? Not funny. It seemed like the comics were, like the rest of the magazine, just excuses to fill one's mind with sex, sexy women, and the promise of their ready availability.

Then there are "artistic spreads," with naked models and lots of interview material which I imagine goes largely unread—childhood hometowns, college studies, aspirations, favorite books…that sort of thing. Pages and pages of pictures, and maybe a little box of text with a few sentences in each.

There were interviews. Dick Cheney was one (one I refused to read, even for your sake, my readers). One was Norman Lear. So it wasn't a left or right thing. Maybe it was an old man thing. There was the "Playboy Advisor" column in which readers (or likely staff writers) wrote in queries, usually about their love lives. Examples: "I really want to take my girlfriend to a strip club: what's the best way to convince her?" Another: "Is it possible for a woman to orgasm just from spanking?" I confess I didn't read the answers: the questions were ridiculous enough.

Then lots of one-pagers on things of male interest like cars, boats, gizmos, and gadgets. All, again, unlikely to be read. Finally, lots of stuff about *Playboy* itself: the culture, the brand, the enterprise. Pictures of Hugh Hefner surrounded by a bevy of bunnies. Pictures of the Playboy Mansion—or one of them: who knows? Smoking jackets. Bunnies. Mansions. Really strange, like a being stuck in a time warp back to the '50s and '60s.

I'm telling you, this is one crazy-ass magazine. It really wants to think of itself as something other than porn. And indeed, it didn't show any sex acts, just women in various states of undress and an overall air of suggestion. But still, the line between this and other less well-regarded magazines (or even websites) is pretty blurry.

7. Raging

The literary review complete, I witnessed something miraculous: I had the most intensely hard erection I think I'd ever experienced. Maybe I was just so awed by having *any* erection that this seemed particularly awesome. But I think objectively that it was bigger, harder, fuller than anything I'd ever had. All in ten minutes: this shot worked wonders.

Kevin came in and asked "how's it going?" I was speechless. He said, "Wow, you seem to be very responsive to the dilation formulation." Really, that's what he said. I had half expected him to burst out into the hall and summon his coworkers: "Hey, everyone, get a load of this: we might have the record breaker here!" But yes, I seem to be very responsive to the dilation formulation. I had a raging boner.

Kevin got down to business. He put a little vibrating rod the size of pencil on my finger and asked me to tell him when I could feel it, turning a dial to raise the level of vibration. I could feel it almost instantly. Sensitive fingers. Then he did the same to my penis. Head, sides, top, bottom. Also very sensitive. He was pleased: no external nerve damage. I was pleased too.

Then he proceeded to cover my newly revived friend with goop and apply a little sensor to various blood vessels on my penis. You could see some screens full of pulsing pings, and others with nothing. Noise. That didn't seem good to me. But I'm not a doctor.

Kevin told me to "hike up my trousers" and wait for the doctor. On his way out the door, he turned back and said, "Oh, the erection ought to go down in about two hours. If it doesn't, give me a call, and we'll see what we can do to reduce it." He gave me his card and left.

8. Testosterone?

A few minutes later the doctor came in. He seemed to remember me a little but spent a few minutes rereading my chart. Then he started talking numbers and results. First, the blood stuff was great. Great flow in. That chart with noise was the flow out: some people have good flow in but during an erection can't keep the blood from flowing out. I had no blood flowing out. Great results, vascularly speaking.

He talked about the virtues of oxygenated blood and how the flaccid (this was a word I heard so many times I lost count) penis rarely gets oxygenated blood. Apparently, for this reason, it's healthy to have erections. He encourages his clients to take a shot every two days even if they're not having sex. Keeps the tissue malleable, healthy. "Really?" I asked. "Every other day?"

He smiled. "I suppose most who take the shot only do it before sex. And that's probably okay too." He said that he'd be glad to set up a meeting with Kevin as soon as possible so he could teach me how to administer the shot myself. I was thrilled. This seemed like a great solution. A hundred times better than Viagra.

Then the conversation got weird (or, if you're not used to talking about this stuff, weirder). He said that I'd had a blood test a few weeks ago, and my testosterone was a little low. My testosterone prior to the surgery had been normal. He said the prostate had the effect of amplifying the testosterone a little. Whatever these numbers meant, I was at 250, and he wanted me to be up at 300—"or even 350."

He thought the lower testosterone might be contributing to the problem of not having good erections with Viagra. He asked if my energy level was good, if I felt like exercising, if I was sleeping well. I admitted that I wasn't exercising as much as I should (or had been) but felt that my energy level was good. My sleep was good, and my sex drive was fine, certainly no worse than it was before the surgery.

Despite these reassurances, he suggested that I consider taking testosterone supplements, at least for a while. They might help rebuild muscle mass (he was looking at my body and wasn't impressed, I guess), increase energy, increase desire to work out, increase libido.

Then he started in on what I call the "medical disclaimer voice." There are two disclaimer voices. The "legal disclaimer voice" is the incredibly rapid voiceover at the end of commercials listing all the things the advertiser refuses to claim responsibility for. The "medical disclaimer voice" is something different. If you ever listen to ads for medications, they usually have someone talk at the end about side effects. But instead of talking through them quickly, they show happy, healthy people biking, blowing out candles, and holding hands on a beach as a calm and friendly voice informs listeners that that product just might turn them into werewolves (or whatever). Testosterone, the doctor informed me with a big friendly smile, might give me acne. Or "cause your hairline to recede a little."

"Anyway," he concluded, "we'll meet in a couple of weeks when you see Kevin. Give it some thought and we'll decide then if you want to. Meantime I suggest you try to work out, maybe eat a lower carb diet. If you don't feel better, maybe you should try the testosterone." Low carb diet? Rebuild muscle mass? I can take a hint. I resolved to start working out like crazy and losing weight. I wanted to come back at the next meeting and say I had exercised and felt great energy. I didn't want to take the testosterone. I'd already had acne once, and I didn't much like it. And my hairline is hanging on by, uh, a thread.

9. Done and not Done

The doctor was pleased that I'd had a good response to the dilation drugs. In case you're wondering, I asked about the suppositories, and he said that they cause aching or burning sensations for most men, so he doesn't recommend them. He didn't look at my erection; I was dressed the whole time. He looked at the clock and saw that I'd had the shot an hour ago. "The erection should be going down soon," he said. "There's a grocery store downstairs; I suggest you walk around, get something to eat. If it doesn't go down by itself, come on back, and we'll take care of it."

So I went down to the grocery and started exploring. My erection was kind of supported by my underwear and pants, so it wasn't too evident, but I needed to walk slowly and with a kind of limp (ironically enough). About thirty minutes into this adventure, I came to a realization: It wasn't going down. It appeared to be getting even bigger.

Yes, even this raging erection, one that seemed to have filled every capillary in the whole member, seemed to be growing even more tight. I went into the bathroom and saw that the head was much darker and that the skin around the penis was completely taut. I worried that it would explode. That's a thing, isn't it?

First I worried about calling for a massive cleanup on aisle twelve. And then I worried about the consequences of having an exploded dick. I limped my way back to the clinic. Everyone was at lunch. So I waited in the office until Kevin came back.

10. Reduction

Finally, two hours after I'd had the shot, Kevin got back and whisked me into the same room we were in before. The *Playboy*s had been put away. He said, "We have two choices for reduction. First, we cut off the whole thing and wait for a new one to grow back." He waited for me to laugh. This is apparently a big joke in the Men's Health Clinic culture. I didn't laugh, though in retrospect it *is* kinda funny.

"Or we give you a shot with a constrictor drug. We gave you a dilator, but it looks like the dose might be too strong. So a shot that constricts your blood vessels should do the trick." So, another shot. And, Kevin indicated, one with a bigger needle.

The shot wasn't so bad. Then Kevin took our relationship to a whole new level. He grabbed my erection and started squeezing it very tightly. "I need to start squeezing the blood out of the penis," he said. "Hope you don't mind." So here I am with a stranger holding my erection and squeezing it. *What if I were gay?* I wondered. *How would that effect this deflation process? What if Kevin were a woman?* The squeezing was pretty intense—and painful.

Eventually, he turned the reins over to me. "Thirty seconds of squeezing, then five seconds of relaxation. It's like milking a cow; you try to push the blood down into the body."

This was very funny, because when I was at camp at sixteen, I remember being taught that milking a cow was "just like stroking your dick." So my life of stroking activities had come full circle. You stroke your dick just like you stroke your dick. Kevin left me alone for ten minutes, and I squeezed as hard as I could and tried to push the blood out. It was really painful, perhaps the most painful of all the things that I experienced that day.

But no luck. Kevin came back and tried it himself some more. He seemed to think the best way to handle a situation in which you are squeezing the blood out of another man's erection was to talk a lot about chemistry.

He talked about various dilation chemicals and the pros and cons of each one. He'd given me a combo of two, one that does a better job of getting the erection but sometimes has this "unfortunate side effect." The other doesn't have the side effect, but it doesn't, by itself, have the same probability of success.

He said that this was all good news, since we knew that these drugs were very effective; we just needed to find the right dosage and mixture to work for me. He said I should think about whether I'd like the combo, but at a lower dose, or the one that didn't cause the current problem but might not give such good results.

At this point, I'd been given two things to think about: Testosterone or no? Combo dilator or single dilator? I wondered why I was being asked for my opinion on these. I am not the professional. I suspected that both my doctor and Kevin had opinions but wanted to give me the illusion of choice.

11. Non-reduction

After about half an hour, Kevin pronounced that the shot wasn't working. I concurred. No progress seemed to be taking place, though it wasn't getting any worse, which was a relief. He suggested we try another shot on the other side.

He also mentioned the "worst-case scenario." My ears perked up. "Sometimes," he said, "these constrictor drugs just don't do the trick. And we need to drain you." I grabbed my erection and started squeezing very hard in hopes of avoiding the draining process, whatever that might be.

We did another shot. Another half hour of squeezing. It went down a little. The skin around the penis was looser. But basically there was still a full erection. We did a third shot. Yes, a fucking third shot of constrictor drug into the shaft of my erect penis. And another thirty minutes of squeezing. But no, this was not working. What went up would not come down.

12. Worst Case Scenario

Kevin went into his supply closet and started frenetically pulling stuff out. Where once the table by my left side was covered with *Playboys*, it now was covered with an array of gauzes, containers, and syringes. He broke out a large jar of mercurochrome and some supersized Q-tips. He said he needed to cover my entire penis with disinfectant. I asked him what, exactly, the procedure was from here. I was imagining leeches. He didn't respond, too busy with his painting project (to which, to his credit, he was devoting great care and concentration). About five minutes later, my penis was completely covered with a brown paint. "No more touching," said Kevin. "We don't want any contaminants at this point." I started to wonder if lasers or radiation was going to be involved.

He said that we should wait for the doctor. Not my doctor, who was busy—too busy for my drainage ceremony!—but the head of the department, a great guy. Kevin went out and then came back in and asked if a new nurse practitioner could watch, a guy named Peter. (Peter? Really? *Playboy* humor seemed to be hitting me from all sides). "Sure," I said. "The more the merrier."

Then the doctor came in. Big, gregarious guy. "Good to meet you. I'm Doctor Johnson." I shook his hand. "That's not really my name, just my profession." He laughed and waited for a little smile from me, which I gave, warily. "Really I'm Doctor Cooper. Nice to meet you."

13. Drainage and Levity

What they needed to do, Doctor Cooper explained, was put a catheter in my penis, a much bigger needle than the previous two models. A "spike," he called it, laughing once more. And then they would pump out the blood, syringe by syringe. He put in the catheter. This one hurt, but once it was in, it was fine. It was a pretty big needle connected to a tube. Peter's job was to keep screwing plastic syringes to the end of the tube and slowly pulling on the end to fill it with blood.

We must have gone through twenty of those little syringes. It didn't hurt, but it was messy: lots of blood spilled whenever Peter would change syringes. Still in training, I guess. I was assured that my groin, which had started to look like a major operating theater, would be cleaned up nice and fresh before we were done.

Then things got interesting. Up until now, everyone had been pretty professional. Maybe it was to cheer me up after having gone through all this. Or maybe it was because it was Friday afternoon. But all of a sudden, Kevin and Dr. Cooper were full of stories and jokes. "I had this one guy, he came to us and had an erection that had lasted forty-eight hours. He didn't want to go to the emergency room, because he didn't trust them. Forty-eight hours! You can do some serious damage in that time. I'll bet he needed a new wardrobe by the time that was over."

"What's the problem with having these long-lasting erections?" I asked, trying to join in on the distraction.

"Oxygenated blood. With an erection, the blood flows in and not out. And after an hour or so, all the oxygen is used up and no reinforcements are coming. So the tissue starts to suffocate. It isn't terrible for four hours. But twenty-four hours? Forty-eight hours? You can really do some damage."

"What kind of damage?"

"The penile tissue can wear down. The walls of the blood vessels can get thin. It can make it harder to get an erection in the future. That kind of thing."

Kevin changed the subject. "So how are your erections lately?" This is the kind of question that I have grown accustomed to strangers asking me. But Kevin and I were hardly strangers by this point.

"Nothing to write home about. My wife and I can get something like intercourse going. But the erection itself? No great shakes."

"That's what we call a stuffy," he said. Peter and Dr. J. laughed. "You just take your penis, form it into a ball, and stuff it in, best you can."

I looked around the office. For the first time I realized it was covered with Viagra swag: calendars, notepads, models of cross-sections of flaccid and engorged penises, and a model showing four kinds of erections: "No erection" (a piece of rubber tubing leaning over); "Some growth, but not enough for intercourse" (a piece of rubber tubing standing up, but easy to knock over); "Erection, able to have intercourse but still soft" (another piece of rubber, standing up but pretty firm); and "Viagra Erection, the full erection ready for successful and satisfying intercourse" (a piece of rubber tubing that I think must have had a steel pipe in the center).

"Yep, you got your stuffies and your stiffies. And your chubbies. You know the difference between a chubby and a stiffy?"

"Nope."

"A chubby is when a guy hasn't had an erection in a very long time and gets one of these shots and gets a little growth and is so thrilled that he has something going on. But it really isn't enough for intercourse. We call that a chubby."

Again, Peter and Doctor Johnson (sorry, Cooper) laughed. "Chubby," they said. This whole junior high drama was all just a way of passing time while the spike in my penis slowly drew out my blood. And it did distract me, I'll admit.

Doctor Cooper stopped laughing. "We're doing two things," he said. "First, we're pulling out the blood that is engorging the penis. But if we just did that, more blood would just come right in. The blood vessels are still dilated. So we're also pumping out the dilation medicine that is still float-ing around and adding in more of the constricting medicine." He pointed to Peter, who was pushing in a clear liquid and then pulling out blood.

I asked Doctor Cooper if having an orgasm would bring the erection down. This was my hard-earned life experience. Though performing the machinations of having an orgasm with this needle in place was far from my mind. "Different systems," he said, somewhat obliquely. "If you get the erection through dilation drugs, the nerve signals of an orgasm don't do a thing."

Finally, after about half an hour, they said that it was time for nature to take its course. They hoped. So Kevin did a little cleanup (lots of blood, as advertised). He covered the area up (catheter still in, but closed off at the end). And they all left.

Maybe twenty minutes later, I looked under the gauze covering and saw that things looked pretty reduced. I didn't want to touch (disinfectant, blood, you know). But I could feel that it wasn't erect any more. Kevin came back in and took out the catheter. Not too painful. He wrapped the whole poor soldier in gauze and tape.

I said, "You know I've had five needles in my penis today? That breaks my previous record by around five."

14. Black and Blue

Before he let me go, Kevin told me a few things. First, he warned me that there was still dilation medicine in my system, and it was possible that things would start to ferment again. If so, I should come back. I eyed the clock on the wall and saw it was three in the afternoon. In a couple of hours, I'd be one of those guys in the emergency room with a boner that wouldn't go down.

Second, he said that I'd be black and blue for a week or two. It wasn't a big deal, just some blood just under the surface that would take a while to get reabsorbed. Already I could see that it was pretty black all over. I tried to make some joke to Amy about "never going back," but she didn't think it was that funny. Maybe she was kind of horrified to see the massive discoloration.

Third, he reminded me that despite all the later drama, the visit had been a big success. I had responded really well (too well) to the dilation shots, and all we needed to do (all!) was get the right dosage. I agree. This was a great day. If I could have an erection even close to the one I had this morning—one that would agree to go down in a timely fashion—I'd be a happy man indeed.

And that's all for now, gentle readers. Signing off. And by the way, though it was nearly all black the next morning, I'm pleased to report that no trips to the ER were required.

Eight Months Out

1. Ding Dong

AROUND NOW, I imagine some of you may be wondering, "I wonder what's up with Marshall's dong?" If you are, please unsubscribe immediately. If not, please read on as though this were as high on your list of topics as it is on mine. It makes it go that much quicker.

There have been a lot of ups and downs in our little saga (starting right in with the artful entendre). Some interesting things to report. Overall I'm in a very good place, perhaps close to a satisfying end place. Yet not quite there.

2. Pharmacology 101

A lot of what follows is about the experience of finding the "right mix" of chemicals to create a reliable erection. If you're not on "team injection" and hoping for progress toward some other modality, you probably will find this one kind of a slog. I'm not saying I've given up on any of the other (less pointy) approaches. Nor am I saying that this one doesn't give a shout-out to them. But mostly, in the last two months, I've been working on the injection stuff.

So let's dive in. There are two functions that allow an erection to occur. One is letting blood flow in. The other is keeping blood from flowing out. Usually these happen at the same time due to what seems like the same mechanism. But they're really two different things. Like two canal locks in different directions.

So, when something goes wrong, the doctors try to find out which is the problem: flow in, or flow out. And there are different drugs for each. Viagra and its buddies (Cialis, Levitra, etc.) are really all about the "flow out" side. As men get older, the diode that keeps blood from flowing out weakens; blood flows in, but it flows right back out. Result: not enough wind to fill the sails. Problems with blood flowing in are less common—for men just getting older, that is. In the prostateless community, not so much. Actually, from what I can glean, it is quite random how the prostatectomy plays out in terms of these problems. Some men are hit in both, some with only one, some not at all.

In my case, it seems to be about the flow in. I have no problem with the flow out. Or rather perhaps I have a different problem with the flow out. I'm too retentive by half. More on this in a bit.

The injection I get is something called a "BiMix," meaning a mix of two different chemicals called papaverine and phentolamine. Now that I look them up on Wikipedia, I see that both claim to be about expanding blood vessels, and both claim to help with ED, by themselves or in tandem. That said, I know my doctor says the second one, phentolamine, is the one that keeps the blood from flowing out. So I'll take his word for it.

The mix (which I order from a special compounding pharmacy in upstate New York) is labeled as "X/Y," which means X milligrams of papaverine and Y milligrams of phentolamine per milliliter of compound. So if I say, "I took 20 ml of 30/0.5," that's what I mean. It's a mixture of these two drugs, and then you take a certain amount of the mixture.

Okay, enough of that.

3. Moving Forward

Last time, I recounted a glorious day full of gore, adventure, and intrigue. The day after that day, undeterred, I made an appointment with the nurse practitioner, Kevin, to learn how to do these injections myself. Kevin suggested I wait a couple of weeks while my weary wand resuscitated. Amazing alliteration, if I may say, and completely unintended. Go figure.

So I went in to see Kevin a few weeks later, all discoloration and discomfort a fading memory. What he'd given me, that first time, was 100 ml of 30/1.0. They weren't really trying to figure out the right mixture for me: they just wanted to make sure I got an erection so they could measure blood flow. Mission accomplished.

But now he wanted to start with a low dose and work my way up. He showed me how to inject (more below) and got the doctor to phone in a prescription for 30/0.5. He said to start with 10 ml and then go up, 10 ml at a time, until I got a good erection—but one that would go down.

4. Injection Instructions

Kevin showed me how to do the injection. There was a lot of general instruction about how to deal with syringes, where to dispose of them, why I should never reuse them, etc. etc. He showed me on two different penis models (models of penises, not men who modeled their penises, though that might be a good career path) where to inject.

If you imagine the penis looking straight ahead (yes, I'm quoting), there is a lot of plumbing underneath. Pipes of various sorts. That is all urinary and ejaculation tubes. Not for injections. On the top, on the left side, and on the right is a lot of tissue. These are the flood chambers. You stick the needle in there, either side, and the chemical flows to all the cells of these chambers. They expand, allowing the blood to flow in. Simple, right?

He gave me a syringe, showed me how to apply an alcohol swab to the jar and the target. Put the syringe in the jar and pull out the right dosage, measuring against the lines on the syringe tube. He told me to inject it in quickly, like a dart. Once in, push the payload in slowly. Then apply pressure to the stab site for about a minute to make sure it isn't bleeding. Then, within about ten minutes, whatever erecting is going to happen will have happened.

I followed his instructions. He watched me do it. He said that I had done it fine. He went away for ten minutes. He came back, and I had to report two things: it came up, and it came down. All in ten minutes. Erection and deconstruction. It reminded me, weirdly, of Jonah and the gourd—alive and then gone in an instant, much whiny grieving on my part.

"That's great," said Kevin. "Means we're on the right track. We just did ten milliliters. Start with twenty, then thirty, and so on until you get the right mix." Seemed like a very sound plan.

5. Home Laboratory

A few days later, the compounding pharmacy called, confirmed a few things (my address and credit card number, mostly) and told me a few things (keep it refrigerated, mostly). The next day, FedEx left a package for me at the door. I would have thought this was the kind of thing that required a signature, but I guess I didn't specify. It was waiting for me when I got home one day after work.

I brought it in and unpacked the box. It had a bunch (twenty or so) of syringes, the kind diabetics use. And wrapped in a foil pouch with some freeze-packs, now melted and room temperature, was a vial much like the one I'd seen in Kevin's office. I put it in the fridge and waited for the weekend.

Saturday morning, we decided to go for it. This was hardly the kind of spontaneity one might ideally want: "Just one second—I need to go to the fridge, get a syringe, inject, grab, and wait ten minutes. Be right back." But God bless her, Amy took this with a proper spirit of scientific experimentation. Masters and Johnson would be so proud.

I did my twenty milliliters. Frankly, it wasn't so bad. Didn't hurt that much, and I felt I did it well. However, after ten minutes, nothing. Nothing at all. This was very surprising, since a few days earlier I had had at least a small and short-lived erection in the office with half the dose. Today, though, nothing doing.

I consulted with my bedmate/lab partner, and we agreed to try another ten milliliters. Still nothing. Then another. Still nothing. Finally, another twenty milliliters. If you're keeping score, that is a total of sixty milliliters, given in four separate injections. But no product.

6. WTF

I pondered my options. What could be going on here? Either:

- There's something wrong with the compound.
- There's something wrong with the way I'm doing it.
- I'm misremembering the previous visit; it really didn't produce an erection in the first place.

I was most inclined to go with number one. After all, the stuff was clearly labeled "keep refrigerated." In fact, another label on the vial said "keep frozen," though Kevin and the people at the pharmacy were pretty clear that refrigeration was all it needed. But it had sat out in the sun for hours. And wasn't cool when I got to it.

I didn't accept number two. I was sure I had done it exactly as we'd done it in the office. It isn't fun, but it isn't that difficult. How can you do it wrong? Miscalculate the dose? I could see the liquid in the syringe. Mistakenly think the needle was in when it wasn't? It was in, believe me. Put it in the wrong place? Nope. I had it staring straight ahead, and I definitely hit the right area. An aside: the doctor later on told me I should alternate sides when injecting so as not to develop scar tissue. Another one of those things I wish I'd heard much earlier on.

And number three was hard to process. Maybe I was making this up? Possible. But I was losing my nerve for more experimentation.

7. Follow-up

I called Kevin and made another appointment for later the following week. I appreciated that he was able to meet with me—they seem to be pretty busy at the men's health clinic. He told me that he thought my hypothesis (that the compound had gone bad because it was out in the sun) was not likely. "The chemicals just don't break down that easily," he said. *So why all the "keep refrigerated" labeling?* I wondered.

He prepared a shot of 30 ml of 30/0.5. He told me to give it to myself. I showed him my (by now well-honed) technique, and he nodded approvingly. He came back after ten minutes: nothing. So he prepared another shot of 30 ml of 30/0.5 and gave it to me himself. "Maybe there's something different between what you do and what I do," he said, searching for a good target point. Ten minutes later, boom: the rock of Gibraltar.

8. We Learn a New Word

At this point, you know the drill. A visit from my good friend, priapism. Pria-what, you say? A new word for us all: priapism. Meaning: an interminable erection. The thing they warn you about with those "four hours or more" commercials. It's apparently a real problem for tissue health, blah, blah, blah. But for me it is mostly a problem of not being about to go outside or even walk. And, as before, it feels like a balloon being filled slowly but steadily from the inside. It hurts.

After he gave me the shot, Kevin told me to "stay nearby" and wait for it to go down. "Call me in an hour if it's still active," he added. An odd word choice: it certainly wasn't active in the sense of getting any. In fact, it seemed completely stagnant. All this talk of blood flow and tissue damage due to lack of oxygen made me feel like I was a walking pool of standing swamp water.

I tried to get dressed and stroll around the local mall, but I was limping like the walking dead and groaning to match. So I just sat myself down in the lobby, nonchalantly crossed my legs, and read through several issues of *Sports Illustrated*.

I must have recrossed my legs a hundred times, and—when people weren't looking—tried to readjust my bundle to a more comfortable or less obtrusive setting. Blessedly, the people in the waiting room seemed as self-absorbed as me.

After an hour, I told the receptionist to call Kevin. He took me back to a different room and had a look at my "progress" (or lack thereof, as it turns out). Ninety minutes, two constriction shots, and lots of painful squeezing later, it was down. No need for the training spike. So there's your good news. But both Kevin and I were left wondering what was going on.

9. Detour into the Land of Three Balls

Before we could dive into our mystery, the doctor came in. He started to go over the numbers around these various shots. He said that there are two critical lines for these injections: the amount you need to get an erection, and the amount that triggers priapism. You want to find a dosage that falls somewhere between these.

But, he said, for some men, the second value is indistinguishable from the first. There is no safe region. "So what's the story for men like that?" I asked, both of us careful not to imply that I might be one of those men.

"In that case, I start to suggest thinking about prosthetics," he said. To his credit, he did not avoid eye contact. Though I might have preferred it if he had.

My immediate image was replacing the defective penis with a new prosthetic one, Steve Austin style. I wondered if I could select the size, thickness, and color. But, of course, that isn't what he meant. He was talking about an implant.

Here's what I gleaned: They put a reservoir of liquid somewhere in your abdomen. Then a balloon in your penis, right where the tissue that fills with blood resides. Then a pump to fill the balloon from the reservoir, and a pump to empty the balloon back into the reservoir.

"So...what's this pump like?" I asked. I'm guessing I'm not the only guy for whom this was the first question.

Kevin jumped in: "It's like a third ball. You squeeze it a few times, and you get an erection. Then you press a little button on it, squeeze a few times, and it's gone."

The doctor continued, "Lots of guys find this preferable to the shots, in fact."

Frankly, I could see that. Though the prospect of another surgery in the groinal region didn't thrill me, it seemed like a pretty simple and clever scheme, given to greater spontaneity than the current one.

However, like the proverbial dick-balloon, my mind was filling. With questions. For example:

- Isn't a third ball something that might creep some people out, like people who are used to greeting two?
- Are there any bragging rights to be had by having three? Is that kind of like having a bigger dick?
- What's with this button? What keeps it from accidentally getting pushed in the throes of passion?
- And what about all this happy talk about oxygen-enriched blood and its virtues for the penile tissue? Sounds like this scheme gives up on this entirely.

So much to ponder about life in Trinadia—that's TRI-NAD-IA. Sounds like a vacation spot, no? However, my doctor's prognostications notwithstanding, it doesn't look like that will be necessary.

10. Mystery Solved

As Kevin was giving me the second shot to bring down the erection, he asked "What's that?" I think I speak for most men when I say that this is not a question you like having asked when someone is pointing at your member.

"What's what?" I responded manfully.

"That bulge. That always been there?"

Sure enough, there was a little lopsided swelling on one side, near where I had done my injection, lo these many hours ago. I felt it, and it wasn't an erectionlike swelling. It was more like a bubble under the surface. Kevin stared at it for a while and poked at it with his finger. "I think this is your injection." It hadn't made it into the penis. It had gone under the skin but not into the tissue.

He went online. The scientist in me liked the intellectual activity I was inspiring. The patient in me—the guy with the injection bubble under his penile-skin—was less enthused. "Yep, I think I know what's going on," he said. "The penis has a membrane under the skin that surrounds all the blood vessels. It protects them from being bruised too easily." I nodded. Of course it does. "I think you may have been pushing the needle in slowly, gradually, and you were pushing the membrane, but not puncturing it. Remember I said you needed to treat it like a dart? I think that's your problem."

This I confess. Rather than jabbing the needle in, I was pushing it in very, very gradually. I think you might understand why. But I can see that this might be the problem and the solution. I asked Kevin what would happen to this bubble of injection under my skin. He said it would get absorbed over the next couple of days. Which it did. Who knows how that works. But it didn't pass the membrane to do it: I think I would have known if it had.

11. Four and a Half Hours

This was very good news. It gave a new lease on life to the injection approach. Ah, but what quantity to use? In retrospect, we should have started from square one: 10 ml of 30/0.5. All my hard-earned data points were invalid. But, for reasons I can't reconstruct, that weekend I decided to go with 30 ml.

To my great credit, I was fine with the dartlike action. And I could feel the difference: it was dramatic. There was a burning sensation up into the head and then back down for about two seconds. Not painful but quite potent. Then gone. I hadn't felt that any of my previous times. I took this as a good sign. And, you'll be pleased to know, the injection worked like a charm.

Three hours later, still mightily engorged, I was resisting Amy's suggestion that we might want to go to the emergency room. When had my life become a scene from some HBO sitcom? But it was painful, and it showed no sign of letting up, so I gingerly put on some extremely loose yoga pants and a sweatshirt and limped to the car.

We went to a local hospital ER, not the place where I'd had the surgery. Thankfully, it was nearly empty. I checked in.

"What seems to be the problem?" asked the intake nurse.

"I, uh, seem to have an erection that won't go down," I half-mumbled, half-whispered.

"Priapism, huh? We get a lot of those on weekends." I wished she wouldn't talk so loud. But I was both comforted and fascinated that this happened a lot. The world of Viagra is also the world of weekend trips to the ER.

We were escorted into a bed secluded by curtains. A nurse came in to interview me and take vitals. I called my doctor. He was on vacation. I left a message on his voicemail, and to his credit he called right back. I could imagine his wife thinking, *Another clown with a boner, ruining my weekend.* He was glad I'd gone to the ER and said I should call him when it was over so we could make plans. I translated this as "third ball."

A resident came in and asked me, "Was it injection, or pills?" So very routine.

He said that the attending would be in shortly and that they'd give me some injections to bring it down. I told him I knew the drill. While I was waiting for the attending, I looked at my watch: it had been over four hours since the injection.

All of a sudden, I realized that my erection was going down. On its own. No injection, no breaking, no reverse milking, no draining. By the time the attending came in, the Hulk was back to Bruce Banner. I was ecstatic. This meant that there really was some space in the region between erection and priapism. The attending came in and asked us to stay for another thirty minutes. Then, nothing having re-arisen, we left.

I called the doctor and told him the good news. He was surprised, but pleased, I think. He said that I was extremely sensitive to the second drug (I withheld sarcastic comments). He said that he'd send me a new prescription with a lower concentration of the second drug—30/0.25. It was non-standard, but no reason they couldn't make it. "Don't forget," he concluded, "start with ten milliliters, and go up ten at a time." I think that part was a little judgy, but I probably deserved it.

12. Square One

As it turned out, Amy and I went into a period of about four weeks in which we didn't see each other—a weird confluence of back-to-back trips. So I told the pharmacy to hold the new prescription until I called them. Then, from the airport on my way home from the last trip, I called them and told them to ship. Got it the next day, and Amy put it right into the fridge. The next day, the science experiments began anew.

13. What 10 ml of 30/0.25 is Like

Nothing. Nothing at all.

14. What 20 ml of 30/0.25 is Like

Imagine Cinderella, in her rags, longing to go to the ball. The fairy godmother casts her spell, and her rags become gowns, her pumpkin becomes a huge and rigid carriage, and she is swept to the ball.

In moments, she is dancing with the prince (I am taking this gender-bending as far as I can without breaking). They are twirling, thrusting, no…not thrusting, uh, waltzing, stepping, pounding, no…not pounding, stay with the story, let's say dipping. Partaking of the thrills of the ball.

But then, just before the climax of the evening—the kiss of true love, let's say—the clock strikes midnight. "No!" Cinderella cries. "A few more minutes!" But alas, she must retreat in haste, the steely carriage reduced to a soft mushy pumpkin.

"Maybe you should use a little more next time," said Amy the prince.

15. Closing for Now

That's where things stand. I think it is all very encouraging. I think we just might find the alchemic concentrations that do the right transformations and reversals. I haven't got it quite right yet. But as the old joke goes:

Q: How do you erect at Carnegie Hall?
A: Practice, practice, practice.

Eleven Months Out

1. On with the Show

Welcome back, my friends, to the show that never ends. I stole that from some old art-rock band, maybe Emerson Lake and Palmer? Still, the show goes on. Ah, but what kind of show is it? Performance Art? Exotic Dance? Political debate?

More and more it feels like a circus. Death-defying sword juggling. Things being shot out of cannons. Beautiful, brave, scantily clad women. Multiple concurrent rings vying for attention. Most of all, of course, we have the delights of the clown car. So much attention on such a (regrettably) small piece of equipment.

A lot has happened since the last installment, but also hardly anything. I'm still searching for the elusive magic potion, the reliable formula. Mostly, I've come out of this last several months with a lot of head banging. If only that were as fun as it sounds.

2. The Life-Force

Sometime around early July, I realized that my libido was suddenly gone. Completely silent, without a trace or echo. I want to linger on this a little. Having had a libido for lo these last forty-plus years, I had never given it much thought. It was an unquestioned part of life, an unquenchable thirst, a yearning inseparable from the yearning for life, adventure, happiness, or any of life's pleasures. Its absence was stunning.

Here's the best I can deconstruct this for you. I think my libido (I can't speak for yours, though if yours can speak, listen carefully) is rooted in a carefully constructed feedback loop. You think about sex. Just like you might think about anything else that comes into your brain. But unlike, say, Angola or Laughing Cow cheese or Uber, a thought about sex triggers fascination, arousal, and then more thoughts about sex. It is self-reinforcing to the extreme, so that the smallest spark of the erotic can incinerate the brain in seconds.

To me, the loss of libido was about the loss of this feedback. Sure, I thought about sex. Mostly, I worried about it, wondering what was happening to it and whether I was going to regain some facility. You see articles about sex on the most respectable of websites, you see sex scenes on TV, it's hard to miss sex triggers. But from there, my mind went... nowhere. Just another thing to enter and leave the stage, like the AFLAC duck.

I even recognized that I wanted to have that excitement and arousal, that I wanted to think more about it, to be fascinated by it. But no—my brain just wouldn't privilege thoughts about sex over any other thoughts. Thanks for writing; we'll get back to you when we can.

I found this very sad. And as I have a few times since beginning this journey, I wondered about chickens and eggs. *Am I depressed, and thus the libido is sunk? Or am I depressed because the libido is sunk?* Or perhaps it was simpler. Perhaps the whole needle-poking thing was so intensely unerotic (for me, at least: I understand that there are people for whom it's a thing) that I had developed an aversion to the whole subject. A general yuck, or anticipatory auugggghhhh.

3. To T or not to T?

All this was on my mind when I had my next visit with my urologist. I asked him about the lack of libido. He asked me a few more questions: Are you having problems reaching orgasm? Uh, sometimes. Are you feeling sad? Not in general, but around this stuff, sure. Are you feeling listless? Yep, hard to get up any desire to exercise. Maybe, he told me, I should consider testosterone enhancement therapy.

I may have mentioned that my testosterone score was around 250, probably down since the prostatectomy, as is common. Not terribly low, but lower than it "should be." Those are his quotes, not mine. He literally said that phrase with air quotes. In Europe, they list the threshold of low testosterone at 300. In the United States, at 350. Why? It's a culture thing.

Frankly I didn't understand what that meant. But then I didn't know what having a testosterone level of 250 or 300 or 350 or even 500 means. How does it change you? He said that he advised many of his middle-aged (screw you!) patients to use testosterone replacement to keep a minimal level. It isn't so much about sexual performance or desire (though, for some, it's about that too) but about what having low testosterone means twenty or thirty years down the road. Decreased muscle mass. Decreased bone density. Weight gain. Lower immunity to various conditions.

I asked him about mood changes—roid rage and all that. He said that the numbers we were talking about wouldn't have any impact on mood or behavior at all. The kind of testosterone-fueled behavior you read about is a) usually not about high testosterone at all or b) about people with incredibly high levels (in the 1000s).

Ordinarily I would have dismissed this suggestion out of hand. I'm not looking for more things to stick in my bulging medicine cabinet. In fact, I called my primary care physician after the meeting and asked him his opinion about all this. He told me that the literature was inconclusive about the effects of testosterone replacement on heart attacks (heart attacks? Who mentioned heart attacks?) but that much of what my urologist was saying was true.

Back at my urologist's, we talked more about sex drive and performance. He said that more testosterone might help with orgasm. And it might help with transmitting the "go" signal. If the nerves are damaged but able to get some signal through, it might amplify. If the nerves are so damaged that they are deaf, no amount of testosterone (or Viagra) is going to help.

I decided to start a small trial: eight weeks. "Are the pills over the counter, or do I need a prescription?" I asked.

He chuckled. This is never something you want to hear coming from your urologist. "No, it's only injected—sorry." It's kept in an oil-based solution, and it's very viscous, so you need two different needles. You use one to draw the stuff out of the jar, and then you replace the needle with a thinner one and use that to inject. I asked him about prescription creams and he said that he felt I needed something longer lasting.

He showed me how to draw the stuff out and inject it. He said to give the injection on the outer half of the upper leg. The outer half has very few nerves; it's mostly muscle, which is where you want to squirt the stuff. The inner half has lots of really important blood vessels, and if you hit one of them puppies, my doctor warned me casually, "you could lose a toe." That really stuck with me: a toe. Not a foot or a leg. Or even multiple toes. I still think of it every time I look for a place to shoot up. Whatever squeamishness I had in the past about needles and self-injection have long faded, given my other shot routine.

So yes, I now have two needle-based routines in my life. At least for now. I will say, though, that the testosterone shots hardly hurt at all. If you choose your spot with luck, you literally don't feel it. Though I am pretty sore the next day on one of my upper legs, outer half.

4. Complex Systems and Multivariate Analysis

I just love that you're still reading after that heading title. But it isn't a joke (at least not entirely). I'm going to throw some crazy data at you; see if you can make some sense of it. It has been three months or so since I've been using the injections of the 30/0.25 mix. Different doses, but the same mix. Over that time, I've had had these results:

Dosage (ml)	Time	Notes
25	4.5	
22	6.5	
15	3.5	
10	3.5	
7	0.5	[1]
8	4.5	
7	2.5	
6	1	[2]
6	1	[2]
6	1	[3]
6	0.5	[4]
10	0.5	[4]
10	7	[5]
6	0.5	[6]

Just so you get your bearings, "dosage" is about how much stuff I put in the syringe. Time is how long it took for the erection to go down. Remember, we're trying to find an amount that will give an erection but not lead to priapism. And notes are, well, notes, described below.

[1] was in the middle of the night, a rarity for us both. How often are we both awake and interested simultaneously at three in the morning? Nothing doing, barely got up, immediately went down, no joy in Mudville.

[2] See how these two look exactly the same? Six milliliters, down in an hour. But the first one was mostly a failure (never that hard, starting to land shortly after liftoff) whereas the second was great (by both accounts). Go figure.

[3] I took Viagra for the first time in many months. My urologist said
     to give it a try to see if it might have some effect. It didn't. So
     then I took a shot. And hardly got any response. But then, like
     an hour later, some erection. Not the usual ten minutes after the
     shot. Made me wonder if the Viagra did something (on its own or
     in tandem with the shot). Calls for more experimentation.

[4] Like a mix of the two in [2]. "Hard but not long," said Amy. She
     meant both temporal and physical extent, alas.

[5] There's a story here, trust me. Be patient.

[6] Tried Viagra again. Really did work this time. About twenty min-
     utes after taking it, a real erection emerged. For about a min-
     ute. Then gone. Then I went with a shot and got pretty mediocre
     results.

Back to the data. What you might notice is that there really isn't any kind of
pattern here. What worked well at one dosage didn't work well some other
time. I was able to go down, considerably, on the dose and mostly avoid
priapism. But down in the six-milliliter range ("that's a really tiny amount,"
per Kevin, my boner coach at the men's health clinic) it is very hit-or-miss.

It makes me ponder two things. First, there must be some other fac-
tors involved. Time of day? Time since recent exercise? Time since eating? What I ate? How long since my last testosterone shot? (I was taking
testosterone through most of these entries, but it builds up in your system, so there was much more in the later than the earlier ones). It could
be any of a million things.

Or, alternatively, it could be that there is variability in the shot itself.
Maybe my injecting skills aren't very regular and I give the shot in such
a way that it gives very different amounts to the floppy recipient despite
drawing the same dose. Or the bottle of bi-mix is getting old and starting
to lose its, ahem, potency—hah! How does that feel, damn vial?

On the other hand, there are lots of variables by which to measure
success. I've been focusing on the boner going down, and thus avoiding

a trip to the ER. But there are many more. Duration of the erection. Hardness of the erection. Length of the erection (weirdly, it sometimes gets hard without getting the full extension). Sensitivity and pleasure. Ability to have orgasm and intensity of orgasm. Plus the whole pain thing (when it is too hard) and the bent thing (haven't had this in a while, not sure what that was or is).

So I'm left with a lot of data, but very little understanding. It still feels like a gamble. Usually it pays off, but sometimes more than others, and sometimes not at all.

5. Pump it Up

I was kind of frustrated and confused about all this. All these shots, all these data points, and nothing becoming more clear, more reliable, more standard. I called Kevin and got an appointment. Here was my thought: if I have a problem with letting the blood in but not with keeping it in, then perhaps I could use a penis pump to get the blood in and use Viagra to keep it in. In my deep scientific understanding of how this all works, it seemed like a good idea.

Kevin wasn't impressed. Two entirely different systems. It always is. The pump doesn't use the nervous system, it just pulls blood straight in without a nerve signal. Viagra only works on amplifying the nerve signal. So no.

"What about the shots and Viagra?" I asked. "Are they playing on the same field?"

"No, the shots are completely different. They don't use the neuro-logical erection mechanism. They're like a back door to open the flood gates when the front door is jammed. They don't work with the front door at all."

"But while you're here, want to try the pump?" I find his positive, adventuresome attitude very heartening. "Sure," I said, "let's give it a roll."

So now I'm going to tell you about penis pumps.

I started asking him about availability. I imagined that I'd have to go to a sex toy shop to get one. I was preparing to tell Amy that she should come with me and stroll among the blow-up dolls, furry handcuffs, vibrators, dildos, leather masks, and sundry unimagined gizmos. Going by myself would make me seem like a creepy perv, but coming in together, we'd be a cool adventurous couple. I think that might have worked.

But Kevin deflated (blow-up doll imagery intended) that idea right away. Insurance used to cover them, but no more. I could get one from Amazon or from a few online suppliers. They run about two hundred dollars.

Anyway, we tried it. I did my part, which was pulling down my pants. Kevin did his. He took the tube (about the size of a large frozen juice can) and put a big rubber flange on the end. He slathered my penis and the surrounding foliage with water-soluble lube. "We need an air-tight seal," he said, shmearing with abandon. Then he put more lube on the open end of the tube and placed my penis inside.

"Push the tube against your pubis so it's tight," he said. And he started to pump the little ball (like the end of blood pressure cuff). After maybe five pumps, he took the rubber flange from the edge of the tube, rolled it onto the bottom of my penis, and removed the tube. This, he told me, was to keep the blood in once the vacuum was removed.

I'll tell you a few things. First, it hurt, and not a small amount. Turns out, the pump isn't in the business of dilating the blood vessels. It just creates a vacuum to get lots of blood flooding into the vessels to the edge of their normal capacity.

Second, the rubber band at the base of the phallus is nothing to write home about. It also hurt a little. But it looked ridiculous. As did the wild jungle of spikey gelled pubic hair surrounding it.

Finally, and this is again about the lack of dilation, the result was a very weak boner. "Stuffable," as the terminology at the clinic goes. But not much more. Not really hard at all.

6. Apples and Oranges

After I got cleaned up, Kevin was in a chatty mood. I asked him about all the different options (shots, pumps, implants, pills) and which were better or worse, more or less popular.

He said, "Well, to be honest, if your original erection is a hundred, none of them gives you a hundred. The implant is the closest, at maybe seventy. The others are more like forty."

"Is that the quality of the erection you're talking about?."

"No, more like popularity," he explained. "Some guys have bad side effects from Viagra or other pills. If it works for them, it works great. But it doesn't work for a lot of guys. Same with the shots. Most guys won't even try them. For those who try it, it doesn't work for a lot of them. But for those for whom it works, it works great, great erection. The implant is a pain because you have to get surgery. Most guys don't want that. That's why I gave it a seventy. But if you get it, most men are happy with it."

"And the pump?" I asked.

"Oh, it's a solution of last resort. Not very popular at all. But better than nothing."

I wanted to take Kevin to task on his scoring scale. In fact, these things aren't comparable. If they work for you, the implant, shot, and pills are good solutions. Nearly as good as the real thing—once you get past the squeamishness, and once you determine it actually works for you. The shot (or pill) is a 100 percent solution for 40 percent of the men. The pump is a 40 percent solution for 100 percent of the men. Not the same thing, but I refrained from bringing this up. In my experience, nerd-splaining is never well received.

7. The Bat Signal

At my next meeting with my urologist (no, I don't meet with him that often, I split the same visit into different sections just to try to make things flow a little better for you) he asked me if I wake up with a morning erection.

I used to, of course. Most men do. Maybe not every morning, but many mornings. I told him no, I did not. But I *did* notice something starting to happen when I started taking testosterone. I would wake up in the middle of the night with the sensation of an erection. It happened several times a week before I could think it was anything other than a dream. I would reach for it, and sure enough—there I was, fishing rod in hand. Occasionally, sitting on the couch in certain positions, I would start to feel myself filling up and engorging. I wasn't sexually aroused; I was just sitting there, perhaps my pants or underwear rubbing in some way I wasn't aware of.

He told me this was great news. Which I was glad to hear. He said that the brain has a pure signal. Brain to penis: "start the erection sequence." Nothing about erotic signals or physical stimulation. Just a pure "go." The brain does that several times during the night, and usually (depending on when you get up in your sleep cycle) when you wake up. It's a way of keeping the tubes in good condition.

In fact, sex provides an imperfect rendering of that signal. You are sexually aroused, mentally or physically, and little-by-little the brain will send garbled versions of that signal. Eventually, it adds up to a true erection, and the signal is coming through loud and clear. But the brain can send the pure thing all by itself. Involuntarily, unfortunately, like a heartbeat.

Here's the thing: There are lots of different kinds of nerve damage that can occur after a prostatectomy. The ability to receive or act on the signal can be impaired. The ability to actually open the pipes and let the blood flow can be impaired too. The fact that I'm having midnight boners means that the signal is getting generated, transmitted, received, and acted on. But in the case of sex, the signal is not very strong. Maybe eventually Viagra will help (as, among other things it serves an amplifier to this signal). He took it as a sign of slow but genuine healing. I will take him at his word.

8. Man Juice, Revisited

No, not that kind of man juice. Which, to remind you, I don't produce—or at least I don't ejaculate anymore. I mean the testosterone. Eight weeks after starting, I went in to my urologist again to review how it was going. The one thing I was sure of was that my libido was back. Pretty immediately and strongly. Plus, my ability to have an orgasm had become much more reliable. So that's something. But other than that, I didn't feel any different. Wasn't feeling more or less energetic. Wasn't sleeping better or worse. Mood the same. "That's interesting," said my urologist. "Because your T-score is kind of high." In fact, it was 960.

You may remember that it had been at 250, and he'd been trying to get it above 350. So 960 would be more. But I literally didn't feel any difference, other than the two not-so-small things noted above. He suggested that I take the shots every ten days and try to reach somewhere in the 600s. I have no idea why 600 is better than 350 or 960. But he did give me a clear indication that my current score was too high. The upside: out of every three weeks, one less injection in my life.

9. Midnight Magic

I promised a story for note [5] above. And a story you shall have. One evening I gave myself a shot at about 6:30 p.m. Usually we are morning people, but we had guests coming for the weekend—long story. Anyway, a good shot, a good erection, a good time had by all. And then, around ten o'clock, I went to sleep. The boner was still strong, but I figured it would go down.

I woke up at one in the morning, and it was still up, harder than ever, and hurting. It had been nearly seven hours. Not good. So I got on a hooded sweatshirt and some extremely loose and forgiving yoga pants, and I drove to the local ER. As you know, I've been there before. Last time, it went down on its own while I lay on the ER bed waiting for a doctor to come by. This time, no such luck.

By one thirty, the doctor was in and said he'd cover me in ice packs and wait until two. If it wasn't down by then, he'd drain. The ice packs were inspired. And a delight. They took my breath away in an instant. But not the blood from my erection. At two in the morning, as promised, the doctor came in. First, a shot or two of lidocaine. That hurt something fierce. But then I was totally numb and totally not watching. So I honestly don't know how many times I was poked. But unlike the previous time at the urologist's office, he didn't fool around with giving me constrictor agents before draining. He was a drainer from the start. Putting in a syringe and pulling out, drawing blood into the syringe tube vacuum. Kind of like the penis pump in reverse, though much bloodier. By the time he was done (some ten or so syringes worth) the erection was down. He then gave me some constrictor shots to keep it down. He said to wait an hour to see if it came back; if it didn't, I could go home. He left, leaving me some towels to clean up.

There was a lot of cleaning up to do. Blood was everywhere: my hospital johnny; my abdomen, groin, and legs; the sheets on the ER bed…I did what I could, but I wasn't entirely clean until I got a shower when I got back home at around 3:30 a.m. Fortunately, the guests didn't arrive until breakfast time.

10. Going out on Top

Well, there you have it. Lots of data, little information. Still hopeful, not quite confident. Pleased with progress to date, but strongly hoping for more. I'll close by pointing out that my testosterone levels are sky-high and yet I remain the same sensitive soul I've always been. To prove it, I challenge any of you to get your testosterone measured and compare it to mine. Loser buys drinks. And go fuck yourself.

Sixteen Months Out

1. Small Wonders

EACH TIME YOU sit to read one of these postings, I imagine you have hopes for some big news, some breakthrough, some V-E-day headline. Believe me, I do too.

But I think we're coming to some stability, with all the comfort and disappointment that this implies. Things are pretty steady and predictable, and many of the riddles have been solved. But the sense that something miraculous still lies ahead is fading. It seems likely that I've reached a new normal, which isn't terrible by any means, but is less than the past normal or the hoped-for future normal.

Of course, by most standards, it is still early. Most doctors say it takes three years to get where you're gonna get. I'm not even a year and a half in. But, data nerd that I am, I can extrapolate trend lines as well as anyone.

Still, read on: this last several months have been filled with enough slapstick comedy, ribald adventure, hard-earned lessons, and emotional alternations to power a small village. Things are good. Some of my sense of well-being comes from genuine improvement. Some, admittedly, comes from lowering the bar a smidge. But good is good, and I'll take it.

2. But I Remember You

About three months ago, I went back for my (slightly past) annual checkup with the oncologist. It was surprising that it had been a year: in some ways, it felt like the surgery was very fresh and recent, in other ways, quite remote.

This meeting wasn't about all the fun and games around sexual function. They had effectively outsourced that topic to the men's health center, you may recall. This was about cancer, a topic I'd pretty much buried in my mind under all the minutiae of injection technique, testosterone levels, and priapism probabilities.

But here I was, back in the same waiting room, signing in with the same admins, sitting on the same couches where I'd been a year before when the threat of prostate cancer and surgery became a sudden reality. Amy had been with me for the previous appointments, but this time I went alone. I thought it would be fairly perfunctory (and in fact, it was). I had been having PSA tests since the surgery, and all had been healthy goose eggs. So I wasn't worried.

Called into the waiting room, I waited for the doctor. In fact, it was Jodi, the nurse practitioner, who came in. I had thought of her often this last year, grateful for the kind words and cautions and patient, careful listening she'd given me.

"Hi," she said, "I'm Jodi."

Really? I thought, *You don't remember me? I'll remember you and the doctor all my days, I assure you.* But I guess I'm just one of hundreds of people who go through this routine.

I imagined that at some point I'd be asked to pull down my pants and expose my scars and penis. "Oh," she might say, "*now* I remember you!" Instead, Jodi looked through my chart to remind herself of the basics. My scores. The nature of the surgery. What the notes said. She looked over the PSA scores and murmured approvingly. She asked about my energy level, my weight, my appetite, my libido. She asked about my continence in a wide range of activities—do you pee when you run? Do you pee when you laugh? do you pee when you sneeze?

Then she asked, kind of generally, about sexual function. Whether I had spontaneous erections (yes, occasionally). Whether I had erections from sexual arousal (no, not really). Whether I had urination with orgasm (yes, regrettably).

I told her I'd been taking the shots and that they'd mostly been working for me. She was pleased. I told her that I was taking testosterone supplements every week to get it up (I'll bet I actually said it that way and didn't even notice. I wonder if she did). She said, "Well, you know that the big risk with testosterone supplements in prostate patients is the recurrence of cancer."

Uh, no. No one had mentioned that to me. Seems like something that might have come up. She elaborated. It isn't that testosterone gives you prostate cancer. It's just that *if* you have some prostate cancer cells floating around, the testosterone will cause them to grow and colonize much more quickly. So…if my PSA score went up, even to 0.1, I was to immediately drop the testosterone supplements and give her a call. "Will do," I said.

"If it comes back," she added almost as an afterthought, "we'll need to start radiation." The whole landscape on which I'd been operating would change dramatically. Overall, however, she was pleased. She said that it was a lot of progress for the first year (some spontaneous erections, some small response from Viagra) and that she hoped more would be recouped in the next couple of years (she's a three-year person: the doctor at the men's health clinic more of a two-year guy).

We talked a little about urination and orgasm. She didn't think there was much to do. Kegels (of course) were always worth trying. There was a PT person she could recommend to help me strengthen my pelvic floor. But mostly it was something that could be improved but not entirely fixed. More on this later.

Time to go. She said the doctor was running an hour behind, but if I wanted to see him, I'd be more than welcome to wait. I decided not to. That way, I could imagine he'd still remember me. (The self-pity is unearned, but genuine).

All in all, I'm glad to have this part of the experience mostly put in the past. All the talk about radiation and testosterone causing "colonies" of prostate cancer cells was more than a little unsettling. And based on nothing, really. I have another meeting with her (them) in a year and then that's it, assuming all is clean with the PSA tests.

3. Spinning Wheels, Got to Go Round

Mostly I'm where we left it. I take shots before sex, and they mostly work. I'm a little stunned at how casually I can talk about it now: yep, I take shots in my penis to get erections. I went past horror to dread to embarrassment to annoyance, and now I've arrived at bland acceptance. I still hope that this is temporary. That some combination of nerve healing, testosterone, and Viagra will lead to a viable alternative. But so far, no such luck. Shots it is.

There are a few things I want to delve into regarding living by the shot. The first is priapism. I still get incidents fairly regularly, or have near-misses. I've spent too much time looking at the clock and feeling my erection: four hours, five…time to go to the ER? Several times the erection has broken (like a fever) in the car on the way to the ER. Once in the waiting room. Once on the examining table.

I've had to go to the ER (by my count) six times. I've thought about going twelve or so. So it is a real concern, and one that is hard to control. Before the erection goes down, there is no sign that it is about to do so. No softening, no change in angle or color. And at five hours, you don't know if it is nearly done or up for the duration.

So let me put it to you. If you had an erection and wanted it to go down, what would you do? How would you manipulate things (the situation, your posture, your endowment) to maximize the chance of de-erection? In my growing anxiety to avoid yet another emergency-room draining, here's what I've tried:

- walking around
- standing still
- sitting down
- lying on my back

- lying on my side
- lying on my front (not for the faint of heart)
- applying a heating pad
- applying an ice pack

Yes, I never understand the whole heat/ice thing, even when I get a bruise. Do I want more blood flowing? That means more can flow out, which is good, but more can flow in, which is bad. Or do I want *less* blood flowing? It's good if less flows in; it's bad if less flows out…I still don't know.

More: I've tried the classic "break it" strategy, which used to work so well in days gone by. But like Bruce Willis, I am unbreakable. Even unbendable. It's a really hard hard-on, much harder than the regular kind. (Though a little bent leeward and shorter, I've been told. So it isn't something to brag about, if that sounded like bragging).

I've tried milking it—that is, stroking it backward from head down to shaft trying to push blood backward out of the erection. Though it sounds like it might be pleasurable, trust me, it is not. Nor, for your future reference, is it effective.

Going for seconds is an option, in theory, save for a few things. Having a perpetual erection, especially after orgasm, is not sexy. Second, it doesn't work, as my advisers have stressed to me over and over. Different systems. The shot puts a chemical directly into the penis, and as long as the chemical is there, it is keeping blood from exiting, orgasm be damned.

I tried standing on my head. I'm not great at this, but leaning against the wall, braced with pillows, I can pull it off. But I get dizzy after a few minutes. And it isn't clear that this even *ought* to work—wouldn't blood be flowing downhill into the penis?

Finally, I think I squared the circle. Here's what I did: I took a long, hot shower. Maybe it worked because it combined the wisdom of the standing still strategy with common-sense advantages of the applying a heating pad strategy. Actually, I have no idea why it works. Nor does it work immediately. But usually within two hours of the shower, the monster is laid low.

4. The Cock Blocker

I mentioned that my erection now is slightly different from the erections I used to get the good old-fashioned way. It is slightly bent to the left, maybe ten degrees, at about midshaft. It is slightly shorter and slimmer, but it's harder. The main difference, however, is the presence of a hard, round mass at the base of the penis, like a quarter or a frozen slice of kiwi. That's what's holding the blood in. It's like a roadblock on an exit ramp. This is the piece that needs to go down. Once it starts to go down—whoosh, it's like water down a drain. I believe that the hot shower thing somehow softens this tissue (or mass of blood vessels, or whatever the hell it is).

I don't think it is visible (not to me, at least). Amy doesn't seem to notice it, though I'm pretty sure she notices the decrease in length and girth…But to me it is the most noticeable difference about these brave new erections I sport.

5. My Life as a John

Let's say that you go to the ER with an episode of priapism. Maybe they drain you; maybe they let you in, and it goes down by itself. Anyway, that's the end of it, right? You go home, tired and happy, and resume your life. But actually, the story ends about four weeks later, when you get a bill. Depending on what they do, it can range from $100 to $400—not chump change, and this is after what insurance covers.

Let's back up a few steps. There was a time in college where I remember being conscious of spending money on condoms. It wasn't much money, but I was always aware of it—how many do I have left? Should I buy the cheaper, or more expensive kind? I was a cheap asshole. Sue me.

Now I'm in a situation where having sex, in addition to the cost of the syringes and medication (a couple hundred dollars a year), carries the possible cost of the priapism. More precisely, the likelihood of priapism (about 10 percent) times the cost.

I don't think about this in deciding whether to have sex. Doesn't enter my mind: I am blessed to be able to afford it. But I can certainly imagine that someone might. It might easily be a factor that kept you from having sex as often as you'd like.

Which brings me to a peculiar set of thoughts. I am paying for sex. I'm not compensating the person with whom I'm having it, true. But I'm enriching pharmacies, syringe manufacturers, ER staff, and, of course, insurance companies. What, exactly, is the line between being a John and my strange situation? Paying for sex is paying for sex.

Suppose we lived in a weird autocratic country where you needed to pay some bureaucratic clerk for a tax stamp in your sex passbook before having sex. Failure to comply would be punishable by, I don't know, fines, prison, some sessions with a dominatrix, or withholding of magic erection-inducing potions. (Note to self: great idea for a short story).

Would paying this tax be as immoral as, say, paying the person providing the sex? I can see that accepting money to have sex is a very complicated moral question. But I open the floor to you: wherein lies the immorality of paying for sex?

6. Nasal Sex

I went to the men's health clinic a few months ago. You may recall that the doctor there put me on a regimen of testosterone shots, and my level went up to 960. So he told me to reduce the dose and come back. My level went down to about 580, which seemed just fine to him. I didn't notice any difference in mood or energy level from the decrease. But I did notice that the frequency of spontaneous erections (during sleep, sitting on the couch) was greatly decreased. It's not that I missed them (it wasn't always convenient, let's just say) but I did like the sense that something was happening in the laboratory.

I asked him whether I'd ever be able to get off the shots. He jumped at the suggestion like he was just waiting for me to ask—which is weird, because isn't getting off the shots something everyone wants? He explained again that there is an erection signal that comes from the brain to the penis during arousal. Testosterone amplifies the signal sent from the brain, and Viagra amplifies the signal picked up by the penis. He suggested that I try Viagra again, but this time he told me to use a short-acting testosterone nasal spray. The testosterone shots are very long-acting: they are slow to build up and slow to break down in the body. But this stuff takes you to "Max T" (his words) in two hours. Together with the Viagra, maybe that would do the trick.

This sounded like a great plan. I was totally excited—though no spontaneous erection ensued, in case you were wondering. This was a show that we could, in theory, take on the road—bringing syringes and refrigerated medication to your average cozy B&B is a little awkward.

Here's what happened, a few days later. Turns out it isn't a spray so much as a gel. You squirt it in your nostrils and then massage it around to make sure the tissue at the back of the nose is coated. You aren't allowed to blow your nose. I coated my nasal passages and took the Viagra, which also seems to take two hours to reach its—and, hopefully, my—max potency.

What does one do for two hours while one waits to be ready for sex? I thought this would be a good time to work out. Get the blood pumping. I wore loose yoga pants just in case things started blossoming. As an aside, I try not to drink any water in the hours before having sex. Fewer problems with urination. So here I am, running on a treadmill, unable to breathe through my nose. Gel was starting to run down out of my nostrils, and my mouth was completely dry from not drinking and from a couple of hours of heavy breathing.

I got home an hour later and was not a sexy, sexy man. My face was covered with snotlike testosterone gel, I was gasping for air, and I was soft as the lord had made me. No amount of stimulation did any good. I was pretty self-conscious about my Neanderthal-like comportment, which might have put a damper on things. We tried this gig a few times and never got so much as a quiver. So back to the shot we go. Maybe we'll try this again when things may have healed a little more. Or so I like to tell myself.

7. A great product idea, and even better name

At my last visit with my urologist at the men's health clinic, I asked him about urination during ejaculation. "What's the big deal?" you might ask. After all, a bodily fluid is a bodily fluid. Sex, if it's done right, involves lots of different fluids intermingling in different ways. What's one more?

That's kind of you. But it bothers me. My continence is completely fine. No problems in nearly a year. No pads, no midnight waking. All good, all dry. Except during orgasm: then I can feel it squirting out, much like my late lamented semen. It is a similar feeling. But I find it embarrassing. Like this is, itself, incontinence. I understand that an orgasm is a powerful muscle spasm and that the usual "hold it in" muscles go lax. Most people have the prostate in between the bladder and the urethra as a dam. Not me, of course.

The urologist gave me a drug to take "a couple of hours" before sex to weaken the bladder spasm without weakening the other spasming going on. I try not to drink water for many hours before sex. I try to urinate like crazy before sex (and often during sex, for good measure). Sometimes these things help. Sometimes they don't.

Back at the men's health clinic, I asked my urologist if there was anything more to do about this. He asked me to urinate and try as hard as possible to empty my bladder completely. Done. Then he did an ultrasound to see if my bladder was, in fact, empty. Sure enough, not empty. He said this was common: after the surgery, there is scar tissue where the bladder was reconnected to the urethra after the prostate is removed. That scar tissue sometimes obstructs the urine from flowing freely. If he were to try to remove some of the scar tissue, though, I'd probably have even more of a problem with urination and orgasm. Or maybe incontinence in general.

I asked, "Well, what's the best way to empty the bladder: standing? sitting?" He told me that it was actually squatting, with the pelvis well below the knees so gravity, as well as the abdominal and pelvic muscles, are pushing on the bladder. Good to know. He gave me the URL for a device called a "Squatty Potty" (I kid you not). You put it on the toilet, and when you sit on it, your knees are forced high up. It's kind of like putting a big stack of phone books on either side of the toilet and resting your feet on them. I declined the purchase. But I do my own version of squatting when I really want to be as empty as I can be. It seems to help. Some. Squatty Potty. Yeesh.

8. Poof: the Magic is Gone

Gel-snot adventure notwithstanding, we had things pretty much down to a science. We had the shot working, I'd learned that a hot shower could help me avoid the ER, and I had some tricks to minimize the urinary stuff. We had weeks, even a couple of months, of pretty regular and satisfying performance.

Then one day I put in the shot, and—nothing. Twenty minutes later (usually I'm up in ten) I put in another shot. Then it was up. This happened the next two times. Then the *second* shot stopped producing results. I had no idea what was going on. I'd been doing this for a while now, and I thought I was pretty good at it. All of a sudden, the magic trick was kaput. And, you may recall, it was really the only decent one in my repertoire. So this was pretty unsettling.

I called Kevin, and we talked over the phone. He said that sometimes you build up a resistance to the medication and need to use more. Maybe double. I told him I was already doing two shots and even that wasn't working now. Plus, I told him, I was afraid of priapism. And would such a change really be so sudden? He went through the basics of good technique: where to inject, how quickly. Yeah, yeah, I was doing all that, I insisted. Something must have changed.

Then I stopped and listened carefully. "Like we discussed," Kevin was saying, "you use a two o'clock angle to insert." This, I swear, I hadn't heard before. Kevin had a standard way of describing the penis as if it were a clock, a comparison rife with potential for lame puns and typos, wherein four to eight were the urinary tubes and eight to four were the blood fields into which to drill. But now he was saying (or I was hearing) something different. It wasn't just the position on the clock, but the angle of the needle. That is, if you're going to two o'clock on the penis, enter in at a two o'clock angle. Otherwise, you're moving down from the blood reservoirs into the urinary area and not breaking the membrane. I don't know: I've been doing the same thing, or so I thought, for a long time. But maybe I had changed it without noticing. Could be, sure.

The next time, I was Captain Timepiece and got my angles completely right. Fifteen milliliters, two o'clock location, two o'clock insertion angle. Why fifteen? I was taking his other advice (double it, plus a little more) as well. So good news: instant boner. Bad news: a trip to the ER. This was one where it faded after checking in, but before being called in from the waiting room, in case you're keeping score.

I found this all surprising and a little embarrassing. I confess that early on I was extremely mindful of the whole process. Lately, I was treating it as somewhat routine. Maybe not giving it the seriousness and focus that needles and penises would seem to summon. Over time, it seems, I was taking my eye off the bat.

But no more: all good for now. Until I get lazy again. Or, say, clocky.

9. Correlation, Causation and Crap

These last six months, I've been working on losing weight and getting in shape. Fortunately, the baseline was so egregious that small efforts are rewarded with big improvements. For a while. Then I tail off and get to a point where it is hard to maintain the routine. I imagine I'm not unique in this regard.

Why am I doing this? My doctors (primary care and urologist) are tag-teaming to give the message that I need to. The primary care doc is talking about long-term risks: I'm actually well within the realm of "fine," but he wanted to make sure I'd be fine at seventy-five. The urologist is talking about improved fitness leading to better sexual function.

So, to the grindstone I go. It has been fine. I'm in a good routine, and so long as nothing throws me off, I can probably sustain it. But I have noticed that over these six months, my blood pressure has been going up: 130, 140, 150, 155, 160 and then, last week, 180—180/110, if you like both numbers. (I'm a systolic guy myself, but hey, there's no accounting for taste).

This is getting into pretty scary territory. I called my primary care physician and came in to talk to him. I confess I was gloating a little as we went in. It seemed obvious to me that the increase was a direct consequence of weight loss and exercise. That I had one of those bodies that really needed to be more prone and puffy. That he had actually damaged my health by pushing this crazy healthiness agenda on me.

We went over all my meds and recent labs. He was surprised. He couldn't quite figure why my blood pressure had been going up. Naturally, he didn't think it was connected to the weight loss. As an aside, he asked, "What did you decide to do about the testosterone supplements?" I remembered that I had talked to him about this just before starting to experiment with them. He had been hesitant and said that the jury was still out on the long-term impact of testosterone supplements. There were lots of small and inconclusive—even contradictory—studies. I decided to go ahead anyway, full of dreams of better erections, increased muscle tone, higher energy, and other manly goodies.

I guess I never told him that I'd started. I told him that I'd been taking supplements and had gone over nine hundred but was now around five hundred. He didn't seem upset that I hadn't coordinated this with him, but he did seem to think it might be related to my high blood pressure. Convenient for him, but it does seem to correlate. During the same six months that I've been elliptical-ing and weight-lifting and experiencing steady blood pressure increases, I've also been injecting testosterone into my outer thighs.

My doctor and I were in agreement: one of these was the obvious cause, and the other was unrelated. We just needed to negotiate about which was which. He ordered some tests (as he is wont to do) to check on other possible causes for the increase, which I thought was sporting of him. Plus he ordered some testosterone labs to get more involved in monitoring the effects of the injections.

Bottom line, if we can't get the blood pressure under control, I may have to go through withdrawal from one of my needle fixes.

10. A Little Perspective

I am nearly fifty-seven. Erections aside, I'm blessed with pretty good health. I realize, though, that entropy is inescapable and that in the coming years it will visit me again and again. I don't know what functions will be impaired, or how severely, or in what order. That's what keeps it interesting—and terrifying.

Some of these losses are sudden and complete, others gradual and—initially—subtle. Some of these losses can be compensated for: different glasses prescriptions, exercise routines, pills, gadgets. Others need to be reckoned with more essentially. Over time, there is a theme of making do with less. Living with diminished capability.

I can take a shot and get an erection for an hour or so when I need it. But there is no shot that you can take when you need to see better for a few minutes, or have clear memory for an hour. There is no pump that steadies your hand from tremors or nasal gel that will loosen the grip of arthritis or paralysis. There is no third-ball implant that can let me stand from a wheelchair when I really want to. As loss of function goes, what I have so far is pretty manageable. Because there are treatments that allow me to recreate the function in some other way, I haven't had to deal with making do without. I've been able to substitute.

To make these shots work, you need much more than just a willing penis and a silenced horrified voice in your head. You need clear eyes, agile steady hands, and a focused mind. If one day I don't have one of those things, the shots will stop being an option. Perhaps my recent two-month stint of not being able to make the shots work was a little foreshadowing of what's to come, someday.

11. Closing

I enjoy writing these posts, and I hope you enjoy reading them. If not, I'm impressed you made it this far! Frankly, I don't know what the future holds. If there are new and interesting developments, crazy or otherwise, I'm eager to share them. The future could look like that: a continued long stream of anecdotes and learning experiences. That's good for the *Boner Report*, but perhaps not so good for me or Amy.

I can also imagine a future that is pretty much like this. Mostly occupying this band of function with small improvements or degradations here and there. That would probably be just fine for me and for Amy, though I should probably let her speak for herself in her companion piece, the Flaccid Report. But it wouldn't be so good for you readers.

It is a dilemma, I'll give you that. I may ask my urologist for more zany treatments or contraptions just so I can report on them. But he may, at some point, not regard his primary role as supporting my particular brand of phallojournalism. So, to the hopeful strains of "Easy to be Hard" from *Hair*, I sign off for now.

Two Years Out

1. For You, the Little People, Who've Made This All Possible

WELCOME BACK TO what I suspect may be our last installment. You've been such patient and loyal readers that I wanted to bestow one last installment before signing off. Because this report has always been all about you. Why do I think this is the last one? Well, read on. But, in short, I think we may be about to tie a ribbon on this whole topic. Which is a shameless transition to our first stop on the erection express.

2. Drip, Drip, Drip

Over the last six months, slow and steady healing has taking place. Small achievements and progress here and there. Nothing dramatic, nor regular and steady. Kind of a two steps forward, one step back kind of thing. But still, taking a perspective over these last several months, definite progress.

The shots are a regular and reliable tool. I no longer worry about priapism, and I have a successful erection nearly every time. When I do not, it is usually cockpit error, as it were—that is, bad injection technique on my part. The erections aren't as good as they were in my youth (or even two years ago): they're a little crooked, thin, less sensitive; I suspect less actual tissue is being exposed due to the diminished expansiveness. But still very functional. Totally okay.

I've been having more success with Viagra too—"more" being relative to "hardly any," of course. But over these last few months, I am seeing more reliable response. The response isn't amazing, but Viagra is now a viable option. The erections are smaller and softer than with the shot, and they are much shorter lived. It takes about ten minutes to achieve erection, and then about fifteen or twenty minutes until they start to wilt. That is enough time for some hanky-panky, but not a lot. I'm also very conscious of this ticking clock, which I'm sure doesn't help.

So I called Kevin at the men's health clinic. He said that I had penile venous leakage. I love that name. Or maybe I love that it is a phenomenon with a name. But basically he's saying that I seem to have no problem getting blood into the penis, but I don't have a reliable mechanism for keeping the blood in. This is not uncommon for men as they get older, prostate or no. You may recall that it looked like my problem was exactly the opposite a year or so ago. I've stopped expecting too much logic from this whole area.

My usual response to this problem is to grab the shaft at the base and squeeze. Much like a half-inflated balloon, this causes all the contents to flow forward, causing a sudden and impressive inflation. But as you can imagine, this isn't a sustainable approach. The minute I remove the hand (which I like to have available for other purposes) the balloon utterly deflates.

So Kevin suggested a penile venous leak loop, something you place at the bottom of your penis as it becomes erect and then tighten so as to keep the blood in. I started on the cheap, as is my wont, by trying a rubber band or hair tie or scrunchie at the base of the penis.

So I tried a variety of rubber bands and hair bands (no scrunchies, actually, they really don't come close to doing the job). Then I went online for the loop products Kevin recommended. If you Google "penile venous leakage loop", you'll see lots of products. Most are more appropriately called "cock rings," which can be purchased in sex shops and, apparently, "make your already big erection gargantuan!" and "Keep you from coming forever!" But they all seem to be based on the same basic idea: you put this ring around the base of your penis, you get some blood in there (your method may vary), and then tighten the ring.

There are only a few problems. First, they don't work worth a damn. Either you make them so tight that the penis becomes purple and numb (two things you never want in a penis), or so loose as to produce no effect on the dread leakage. And second…

3. Adventures in Manscaping

Getting a rubber band entangled in a thicket of pubic hair can be downright painful. That seems like a pretty obvious statement, but it wasn't obvious to me at the time. Each time I'd wrap the band around the base of my penis to try to keep blood from flowing out, it would require many minutes of gently trying to disentangle the band from the jungle in order to remove it. I'd emerge from the struggle with the hairs pulled every which way and the shaft skin rubbed raw.

So I decided it was time for some deforestation. I figured that if I had no pubic hairs, the seal of the band would be tighter and the effort to remove it less arduous. I don't know about you, but I've never had any care regimen for my pubes. I never combed them, trimmed them, or slathered them with conditioner. They were pretty self-sufficient. So I didn't know exactly how to go about this. The idea of shaving that area (including all the hair on the base of my shaft itself: is that normal?) was very unappetizing. I wondered if this is something professionals do for you, but the application of hot wax and rapid yanking sounded even worse.

So I went old-school, scissors in hand. I guess I've gotten pretty cavalier about having my privates in proximity to sharp objects. It took a surprising amount of time, not due to my extremely dense mop of hair (I think it is pretty moderate, to be honest) but to the cautious, plodding manner I took. A few hairs at a time, separated from the herd and snipped down.

By the end, it was a sight to behold. I hadn't seen my penis without hair since junior high, and there wasn't much to behold back then (though I should have taken pictures just so I could gloat on the progress in the interim). I can't say it was a beautiful thing. The penis is, after all, kind of a weird-looking contraption, and removing its coat doesn't make it any less so.

To the question you're no doubt asking—"well, did a hairless johnson help with using the rubber band?"—I'd say yes and no. It didn't really help with the erection. But it made it a lot easier to remove after the failed attempt. So that's something.

4. Shhh...Do not Disturb

One thing about Viagra erections (or any half-baked erection I can occasionally summon into being by manual means) is that they are extremely temperamental. They can collapse at any moment, like a soufflé. And, as with a soufflé, you tend to whisper or tiptoe around trying not to disturb the poor thing. Which is not a great atmosphere for the lovemaking.

It's an odd thing. It's like having a third party in the mix, and not in a wild, ménage à trois kind of way. There's me. There's Amy. And there's this spoiled prima donna who may deign to participate in our little party, may snub us entirely, or may show up drunk and collapse on the couch asleep.

5. Groundhog Day

OK, I confess: I keep a journal of our sex life. I didn't used to: it isn't some kinky thing I like to refer to for future arousal like a sex tape. It's something I've been keeping these last two years to monitor progress, or lack thereof: what we tried when, how it went, and so on. It is like the most boring letter to *Penthouse Forum* you can imagine.

Mostly I just write these entries and ignore them. But when I'm about to sit and write one of these reports, I review all the entries since the last report. Here's the funny thing. In the last six months, there are at least six entries that read something like:

Hooray! Milestone! Amy and I had successful sex without a shot! This is <u>real progress</u>!

Each time, I'd write it again as though this was the first time it had happened. This is very hard to figure out. Why did I have no memory of it having happened before? It's a puzzler. But, of course, I have a few theories. First, sex is very much an in-the-moment thing. It is often hard to recall what happened hours, let alone days, later. It is very intense (if you're lucky), and as the body fully engages, the mind disengages. There's only so much blood to go around, after all. So it isn't that surprising that such a momentous moment could just not register.

Second, I think there's some underlying restlessness or perhaps false enthusiasm in these notes. (Witness the underlines and overuse of exclamations.) Each time is an achievement, to be sure, but perhaps it doesn't feel quite as great as the moment should feel (there's that underline instinct again). So the words get captured, but the sentiments slip away.

Finally, having sex without the shot has been hit-or-miss. It has failed as much as it has succeeded. So the memory of the intervening weeks (with a shot or two successfully executed and a non-shot less so) may do a lot to erase the achievement of several weeks before.

6. Scheduling Conflict

I have found my performance on Viagra underwhelming, to say the least. It doesn't get very engorged, nor does it stay that way very long. Why is that? Sometimes, maybe once or twice a week, I wake up in the middle of the night greeted by a really substantial boner (mine, in case you were wondering). So what's the deal? Why can't Viagra do something similar?

A little background: First, I've been taking my testosterone shots every Saturday night. (Turns out the blood pressure spike had nothing to do with the testosterone, and has since been taken care of by some new, unpronounceable pill.) My Penis Team tells me it needs to be at a regular time, but it doesn't matter when. So I started Saturday night and have stuck with it for this last year.

Second, Amy and I have sex pretty much every Saturday morning. Not *every* Saturday morning. And not *only* Saturday morning. We're not robots. But that's our habit. More on this in a bit.

You are probably way ahead of me. But it literally took me months of pondering to figure this out. Not enough blood flowing to the brain these days, I guess. Taking testosterone shots Saturday night means I am at "MAX T" a couple of days after that, say Tuesday or so. Saturday morning would be, wait, let me break out my slide rule, "MIN T," literally the lowest level of testosterone my body has. These midnight erections I've been having (yes, I've kept a list, you know me too well) have mostly been on Mondays, Tuesdays, Wednesdays. The occasional Sunday or Thursday. Friday and Saturday, never.

Long story short, I moved my shot schedule to Wednesday night. Has it helped? Yes, I think so. The Viagra has at least been more predictable. I still have the leakage problem, which I don't think Viagra alone can fix. So I'm still experimenting with the loop. But it is definitely better. And, to top it off, I'm finding the orgasms to be much more intense, and certainly more intense than with the shot. This is odd, since the shot makes all the penis tissue taut and exposed for stimulation, whereas the Viagra exposes a smaller surface area. Then again, the orgasm takes a lot longer to build and achieve. So maybe it is the greater testosterone level, or maybe it is the slow gradual build. But it is pretty wondrous.

7. The Great British Boning Show

Amy and I saw a show the other day talking about kitchen life in Britain during World War II. Everything was rationed. You could hardly get anything you would normally want to cook or bake with. No eggs, no flour, no sugar. Everyone was encouraged to subsist on what they could magically conjure from their backyard gardens. This had a big impact on domestic life. Before the war, wives were used to being able to create great dinners and desserts for their husbands and children. These same husbands and children were used to receiving them. Compliments were given and received, and everyone felt great.

But during the war, the meals were incredibly meager, low in nutrition, and unappetizing. The newspapers were filled with recipes for "mock" everything. Take, for example, mock peach pie. You would make a crust out of mashed potatoes and a filling out of beets. If you kept a few bees or a honeysuckle bush out back, you could add a little sweetener. But you can imagine that the mock peach pie didn't look or taste anything like actual peach pie. Back to the domestic scene. The wives felt inadequate. The husbands and kids were disappointed. Perhaps compliments were given and received, but everyone knew they were just to mask genuine feelings.

But here's the thing. The war went on for a long time. Over time, the families started to develop a great appreciation for the hard and creative work the wives put into creating these meals and desserts out of limited and unconventional ingredients. The wives started to feel proud of their achievements. And tastes changed. Mock Peach Pie started to taste, if not like actual peach pie (the remembered taste of which was starting to fade), but like something enjoyable in its own right. What were once forced compliments and pride became real compliments and real pride. Amy and I watched this show and found it very moving.

8. Regularity to Ritual

Careful and snarky readers may have noticed the comment above about a regular Saturday morning schedule and thought, "Jeez, where's the spontaneity? Your sex life has all the spark of changing the fire alarm battery."

To which I might reply, "Fuck off." But then, thinking better of it, I might reply like this: Before this surgery our sex life was unscheduled. Of course it was. Whose is? Really, I want to know. And that lack of regularity carried with it this unspoken tension. Two people need to overlap their desires for this to work, or at least work well. I spent a lot of mental energy wondering when we'd have sex.

Then the questions of "how" and "whether" overtook everything. The ability to actually perform adequately has been so unpredictable. Of course, here and on nearly every page of this journal, I need to express my love and gratitude to Amy, and I will in a few pages. But to put it briefly, she took *when* off the table and allowed us to focus, together, on the *how*. She turned a problem into a project, and then together we imbued it with the power of ritual. So we can feel we are doing and (gradually) accomplishing something together. We can exchange high-fives, review the results, plan next steps. It is a kind of intimacy that I don't think I've ever experienced, let alone associated with sex.

Sex is a wonderful thing. And our sex life is very different from what it was even two years ago. Back then, we had the full menu available from which to pick and choose. But really, didn't we usually pick the same handful of things from this sumptuous menu? Don't most couples? Now we have an extremely narrow menu, like one of those hand-written affairs you get at small pretentious bistros. But we order the whole menu.

So I wouldn't say it is worse, by any stretch. It is full of meaning, of love, of gratitude, of adventure. And that is not something I thought I'd be saying a couple of years ago.

9. To Shoot or not to Shoot?

Okay, we now have two essential erection delivery systems. The BiMix injection, and Viagra. I also have a few Cialis lying around that I might try some time, but it's largely the same idea. We tried pumps, testosterone gels, and loops, and they brought more trouble than they were worth. So these are the two.

Which is better? When I choose—usually Amy is pretty open to gambling on whatever number I feel like playing—what goes into the choice?

A debate between pros and cons is what the situation demands. First, the shot:

Pro: It is tried and true. Nearly always works.
Con: Yep, nearly always, but not always. Also, do I have to remind you? It involves sticking a needle in my penis.

Pro: But I've gotten used to it. Hardly ever hurts.

Con: Yes, but I'm starting to get scar tissue from the injections. My penis sometimes feels like a sack of rice, and not in a good way.

Pro: When you inject in a scar tissue area, it doesn't hurt at all.

Con: But it also doesn't work when you hit scar tissue. You basically have to poke around, like an addict trying to find a vein between his toes, until it hurts. That's how you know you've avoided scar tissue.

Pro: Enough of this. The erection is rock hard.

Con: Yes, but it's skinny and bent.

Pro: It allows for a greater variety of positions.

Con: In theory, but the skinny and bent thing is kind of limiting.

Pro: The erection usually lasts for an hour or more.

Con: Thank god the fear of priapism has receded. But still, you can't go outside for an hour after sex, and mostly need to wander around in yoga pants.

Now, the pill:

Pro: Easy to take, duh.

Con: Can't argue with that. It is kind of expensive.

Pro: You're so cheap. I refuse to even continue this debate.

Con: Sorry, I take it back. How about "The erection is short-lived"?

Pro: Fair enough.

Con: Nothing to write home about, firmness-wise.

Pro: No argument there either.

Con: It takes about ten minutes for it to start working, and another twenty minutes later it's gone. That's a pretty narrow window in which to try to please the missus.

Pro: The loop really does help with both duration and inflexibility.

Con: True, but it's an awkward thing that needs to be adjusted
      a lot. Too tight or too loose is not a winning formula.
Pro: The orgasms are often very strong.
Con: If you can get it in. Sometimes it is like trying to insert
      Jell-O into an electric socket.

I'll let them fight it out some more. It is unresolved, but I'm still hoping for some great improvement on the Viagra front to tip the scales. That said, I'm just glad to have two (even imperfect) solutions to fight over.

10. Biennial, Semiannual...Whichever the Hell One Means "every other year"

I have an appointment in a few weeks with the urologist/oncologist who performed the surgery two years ago. This will be my last meeting with him, barring some highly undesirable movement in the PSA index. I expect it will be a short and drama-free visit.

So much has happened these two years that it is hard to put myself back in that office when the diagnosis was given and digested, the options were being discussed, the consequences absorbed. Many people have come up to me recently and said, "Hey, congratulations! Two years! That's a big deal!" I confess I have been kind of taken aback each time it has happened. Who knew that people kept track of how long it had been since I'd had the surgery?

Two years of straight zeros on the PSA score is a pretty good indication (though eternal vigilance, blah, blah) that they got the devil in its entirety before it spread. So it is very encouraging. But I realized how little I've been concentrating on the cancer. As you know, I've been focused on this tale of willy woes and all its comic twists and turns. Were it not for all this ruler-in-hand self-absorption, I'm sure I'd be in continual freak-out about whether this or that ping was a resurgence of the cancer. It has been the most wonderful distraction.

Three Years Out

1. This Time For Real

A YEAR AGO, I put together what I thought would be the last installment of this little serial. It seemed like there wasn't likely to be too much more to write, and things had reached a kind of plateau. But here we are, one more year along and I've gathered, if not wisdom, at least some more anecdotes and updates. I've also started to think of compiling all these tidbits into one big collection, which brings on its own set of puzzles.

This is the last installment, I promise. So please read on, you're in the home stretch.

2. I Heed Some Good Advice

Careful readers might have noticed something funny as they made their way through these pages. The book cover calls this *The Bone Reporter*. But inside the cover, I've been calling it the *Boner Report*. What gives? Good catch. In my head, I've always been calling this little journal *The Boner Report*. Like a Wall Street ticker tape, or a real-time chyron of my ups and downs.

Then I went to a prospective agent and asked whether there might be a market for ramblings like these. His immediate response was, "You gotta change the name."

"Why?" I asked, genuinely surprised and a little disappointed.

"Well, if you want people to find your book online, and they type in the name and they get porn, that's not a good name."

Sure enough, if you Google "Boner Report", you don't, alas, get this book. No, you get several podcasts and related blogs and websites. All, it seems, dedicated to reviewing various sexual conquests. Honestly, I'm not sure: I didn't subscribe.

So *The Boner Report* had to go. I decided to keep the title inside the covers but put a brown paper wrapper of a title on the cover. I spent more time than you'd think would be needed to come up with an alternative. I spent a few hours or days living with each of these:

- *The Re-Erector Set*
- *The Resurrection Project*
- *The Potency Report*
- *Ain't It Hard*
- *101 Recipes You Can Make with Ground Sausage*

Finally, I settled on this one. It keeps the spirit of the original alive with slight hints of forensic journalism mixed in. Plus, as of this writing, you can type it in and get no porn.

3. AKA

Having corrupted the name of the book, the thought occurred to me try out a pseudonym. It might be fun. It would preserve privacy. It would provide an opportunity to buy back a little of the zip I lost with the title.

Here are a few I considered that I think reflect the right spirit:

- Rob Peterson
- Flaccido Domingo
- Peter Droopman
- Dick Dastardly

Finally, I decided against it. One thing you need is an assurance that this is all real. If I read this and found out later that it was fictional, I'd be pretty pissed. The author's name underwrites the authenticity.

So here it is, signed by my own hand.

4. Maybe Prone Would be Better?

I've learned two things about the word prostate in the last several years. First, no one seems to be able to tell it from prostrate. Prostate, prostrate. See the difference? There's a second "r."

Whenever the word prostrate comes up (which it doesn't that often, admittedly), people tend to say something like "He was lying prostate." And then correct themselves, "I meant prostrate. Wait, which is which?"

The second thing I learned is that I am now the proud owner of this word. After these verbal stumbles, someone inevitably turns to me and says "Sorry." Like I'm the goddamn usage police. People hear "prostate," they think me. There's an association to be proud of. It is a little surprising because it has been a long time, and I'd assumed that my brush with prostate notoriety had faded. But no. I'm the go-to guy, prostate-wise.

5. In Desperate Search for a Mnemonic

The venous loop that I use to trap blood in my aspiring wang is a thin rubber tube with a plastic fastener that keeps it in a noose shape. On each end of the tube is another fastener that you pull on to make it tighter or looser. You open the thing up to max looseness, put your penis in, and then pull on the tightener until it feels right. Good enough.

Here's my problem. On one end is a round ball. This one says, "Loosen Me." On the other end is a flat disk. This one says, "Tighten Me." In the throes of passion, and no little desperation, I never remember which is which. I have tried for over a year now to come up with something that I can remember, and nothing. This is no small issue. When you put it on, you tighten it, and then you may need to do some adjustments midstream. You start to feel a little numb (a tingling, but not the good kind), and it needs to be looser. The erection isn't quite keeping up, and it needs to be tighter. You have to pee in the midst of things, and it needs to be a *lot* looser. In any of these circumstances, if you make the wrong choice, it can be pretty bad: lots of pain, or lots of blood loss (internal, that is). So it would be good if I could remember which was which. But usually I just pick one at random and see what it does. Not a great system, I'll admit.

The problem is that it doesn't make sense. Flat should mean "deFlate." Round should mean "Ready." Flat should mean "Squashed." Round should mean "Full." Any of those would be great. I could remember that. But it is just the opposite.

By the way, if you have a mnemonic that says "Do the opposite of what you think it should be," it doesn't go well, trust me—"is that what I think it should be? Or is that already after I've flipped it? Oops, we're down…" I have written a constructive yet stern letter to the venous loop company, but haven't heard back.

6. Signals Crossed, Again

I had an appointment at the men's health clinic a while back, my first in many months. Mostly all is fine. Testosterone levels good, libido fine. PSA score flatlined. The conversation quickly turned, as it will, to erections. The doctor asked about how things were going and what I was doing. I told him that I took the shot and it mostly worked. But once every three or four weeks I'd try a Cialis before sex and have underwhelming results. Sometimes adequate with the loop, never without it.

He seemed puzzled. Not that I wasn't having good results. That happens. The "try a Cialis before sex" part. "Aren't you taking it daily?" he asked.

"No, why would I?"

He had given me a prescription for Cialis many months ago. I got a bottle of ninety of them. I figured, "great, this will last me for a couple of years!" But his intent was that I take one every day. He could swear he'd made this clear to me. This must be the millionth time they've said something and I've missed it because I was spacing out, distracted, whatever.

I asked him what the point was of taking one every day.

One word: Vascularization.

Cialis increases blood flow to the penis tissue. It is a more focused, newer drug than Viagra, which increases blood flow to a whole class of tissues. That's why Viagra sometimes causes seeing colors or spots, headaches, and a few other symptoms.

Keeping the penis tissue awash with oxygenated blood—vascularized—could help with tissue regrowth and healing. He said that while we'd been focusing on nerve damage and healing, the health of the penis tissue was also something that needed to be cared for.

I wondered about the impact of having Cialis constantly swimming around in me. Would I be in a constant state of arousal? More prone to side effects? What would be the impact on blood pressure? Given the low dose, he didn't think there would be any.

That brought up another point. The daily dose is relatively low, seven milligrams. For a one-time in-time-moment dose, it is low (usually people use fifteen or twenty). For daily, it isn't so low. Some people take it daily at five or less. But for me, two something years out from prostate surgery, he wanted to go with seven.

He said to consider the daily Cialis as an addition to whatever was done at the time of sex. Take Viagra. Take the shot. It should help with those as well. Maybe the daily Cialis itself would help on its own—we'd see, give it time.

7. Life with Constant Vascularization

So what is it like taking Cialis every day? In general, I didn't find that it made much of a noticeable difference. No change in blood pressure. No headaches or lightheadedness. No spontaneous, uncontrollable erections, sadly. But it is true that my penis is continually more filled with blood. A tiny bit. Not something you feel. It isn't aroused. But occasionally, when I pee, I can look down and say *"niiicce!"* Has it helped with sex? I think so. The erections with the shot are slightly better, and those with Viagra are considerably better. So it is definitely helping on that front.

8. Taking a Final Stock

When I woke up from surgery and saw my oncologist and nurse there, they first invoked the magic of "three years." You only know where you're going to get after three years. It is still early: you have three years. It takes up to three years for that to come back, if ever. Well, here it is. Three years, almost to the day. So if I only know where I'm going to get after three years, where have I gotten? What do I know?

- My PSA score has been zero for the last three years.
- My scars have disappeared to the point that I can't even find them.
- My urinary continence is completely fine. But I do often urinate when I orgasm.
- I take weekly testosterone shots. There are a lot of reasons why this might be a good thing, but the most tangible is that my libido collapses without it.
- I cannot get an erection without help from medicine. I do get night erections occasionally, though not often.
- I take shots to get erections. I no longer think there's anything odd about giving the shot and don't flinch at the thought. I have figured out dosing so that I no longer get priapism.
- I take Viagra to have sex as well. It doesn't work as well as the shots but is *much* more convenient. To really make this work, I need to wrap a rubber tube tightly around my penis to help it retain blood. To make *that* work, I need to shave my pubic hair periodically.
- I take Cialis daily. It leaves me in a constant state of extremely mild engorgement and enables somewhat better erections with the shots or Viagra.
- My sex life with Amy is still a great source of joy in my life, maybe more than ever.

If I had seen that three-year report sitting there in my hospital, I know I'd have been pretty pleased. Relieved. And yes, three years later, I am.

9. This is Predicated on the One I Love

With that I'll sign off. I can imagine some reason for a future update, but I can more easily see that there will be no more reason for an update. Just straight ahead, we can only hope. In the unlikely case that this set of words ever gets to a point where it needs a dedication, I've been trying out a few. Here's my best, let me know what you think:

For Amy[1], because you can't spell "My hard-on" without A-M-Y.

---

1 About whom, words fail. She has made this terrifying prospect into an exciting adventure. She has provided the most rich and enduring patience, resilience, and confidence precisely when mine flagged. She has taught me something about love and intimacy that I never had a clue about before, and this after thirty-something years of a loving marriage. She has been a fount of good humor in what has often been a dreary business, and a fount of perspective where memory and context are hard to access. I am in awe, I am in love, I am awash in gratitude. Plus, awesome mock peach pie.

www.ingramcontent.com/pod-product-compliance
Lightning Source LLC
Chambersburg PA
CBHW070838260726
48660CB00005B/2082